The Lives of Foster Carers

There are approximately 37,000 foster families currently living in the UK, yet while there has been a substantial amount of social research about fostered children, little is known about the adults who look after them. By focusing on the carer, not the child or the social worker, *The Lives of Foster Carers* offers the reader a new perspective on foster care. It explores the contradictions, conflicts and ambiguities faced by foster carers every day and looks at how public bureaucracy and private family life intertwine. The issues it discusses include:

- a history of the foster care service
- professionalising foster care and the shift away from foster parenting
- public and private domains in foster care
- motivations and roles of foster carers
- how foster carers perceive themselves and their foster children.

Based on a wide range of literature and in-depth interviews with 46 foster carers, this book provides valuable insight into the concerns, processes and experiences of foster carers. Jargon free and accessible, it will appeal to foster carers, practitioners, students and academics in social care, youth work and child care as well as policy makers in children's services.

Linda Nutt is a foster care and child-care consultant.

The Lives of Foster Carers

Private sacrifices, public restrictions

Linda Nutt

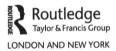
Routledge
Taylor & Francis Group

LONDON AND NEW YORK

First published 2006 by Routledge
2 Park Square, Milton Park, Abingdon, Oxon OX14 4RN

Simultaneously published in the USA and Canada
by Routledge
711 Third Avenue, New York, NY 10017

*Routledge is an imprint of the Taylor & Francis Group,
an informa business*

© 2006 Linda Nutt

Typeset in Times by BC Typesetting Ltd, Bristol BS31 1NZ

British Library Cataloguing in Publication Data
A catalogue record for this book is available from the British Library

Library of Congress Cataloging in Publication Data
A catalog record has been requested for this book

ISBN10: 0–415–35811–6 (hbk)
ISBN10: 0–415–35812–4 (pbk)
ISBN10: 0–203–00412–4 (ebk)

ISBN13: 978–0–415–35811–8 (hbk)
ISBN13: 978–0–415–35812–5 (pbk)
ISBN13: 978–0–203–00412–8 (ebk)

To Mark and Susie who looked after me for two whole years and showed me new hope in ways of the world.

With love from Bryan

Dictated by Bryan, aged 12 years, who was in foster care from two until he was four years old.

Contents

Introduction

At any given time in the UK over 70,000 children are in public care, the majority of them living with foster families.[1] Despite the importance of this service, qualitative research focusing on the foster carers is scant. We know little about their day-to-day lives and how they manage its bureaucratic context; how they cope with the problems and the challenges that they face.

The Fostering Network's[2] annual review for 2004 states that 74 per cent of the children in public care are living with some 37,000 foster families, which they estimate to be about 10,000 too few. The majority of foster families are registered with local authorities. There are also a number of independent fostering providers (IFPs) in the UK but they are outside the scope of this book. This book explores the world of local authority foster carers; at how they construct themselves and their lives. It does not include other perspectives: those of the fostered children, their families or of the social services. Clearly these alternative frames of reference and important dimensions would help to more fully appreciate the foster carers' position, but this research is solely concerned with foster care from the perception of the adult carers, in contemporary society, with a particular focus on the UK context.

Using the available research together with new material from in-depth interviews with foster carers, this study focuses on their little-known and changing world in order to give a broader understanding of their family lives. The 46 carers (see Appendix A) represent different nationalities, cultures and class whilst including all types of local authority fostering from emergency placements to 'quasi-adoption'. They include a full range of ages, lifestyles, geographical areas, own family constitutions and single carers of both genders. The interviews concentrate upon their lives and their understandings and not upon the foster children as there already exists an extensive body of research work about them. Nonetheless, analysis of the scripts finds that life-as-foster-carer is centred on and around the children.

It is known that not all carers provide a quality service; there are many where the social services' perception is that the children's care is substandard. Official reports identify the potential for negligent care and actual abuse (Waterhouse, 2000; Utting, 1997; Berridge and Cleaver, 1987). Ward and colleagues' interviews of children in foster care (2005) give examples of children who were discriminated against and felt excluded. Virtually nothing of this is evident in this examination. A different analysis of the study carers might have uncovered hints and generally this study would have been more complete had it included some foster families where a disparate commitment had produced contrasting data. It is not possible to tell whether there are any such carers in this study, only to note that generally in interview respondents manage self-presentation, and research shows that parents wish to appear competent and adequate (Baruch, 1981). The study carers are no different.

The study foster carers portray themselves as dedicated to the children that they look after. They present a preferred, possibly over-positive version which may read as uncritical. This is perhaps because their accounts are for the researcher as 'public' audience. Additionally, prohibitions regarding the chastisement of children in public care may pressure them into rationalising the children's behaviour. One of the purposes of the vignettes (Appendix B) was to note whether the carers, who might take a normative line in interview, would perhaps reveal a difference in personal practice. A search for diversity, possibly because of fostering experience or ethnicity or gender, has not demonstrated dissimilarity of perspective. The striking feature is that, although the carers are a diverse, heterogeneous group, their views, experiences and constructions are consistent across interviews – foster children are their priority.

The names of all research participants, their foster children, individuals mentioned by them and any locations have been changed for reasons of confidentiality. The foster carers were all invited to choose their own pseudonym.

1 What do we know about foster carers?

The applied social research

Foster families and their homes are the favoured option and primary location for the delivery of service for children looked after by the local authority. Yet as Berridge (1997) identifies, the foster care service remains under-theorised whilst Sinclair and colleagues note that, although most UK councils have special fostering schemes for teenagers, they 'typically lack the elaborate justifications of their North American counterparts' (2004: 9).

To set the context for an analysis of the foster carer world, this chapter reviews the social research literature on foster care with particular focus on the carers themselves. Included is a brief outline of social policy pertinent to child care, plus a short history of the growth of foster care as a resource for looking after other people's children. A background description explains how the foster care service is situated within local authorities, with some information on the several administrative classifications of carers. The chapter also reviews what is known about the characteristics of foster carers and concludes by looking at the literature that seeks to faithfully reflect the foster carers' own views, perceptions and explanations about how they make sense of their role. Overall it summarises the current social research knowledge about the foster carer's environment.

There is a close connection between the histories of childhood and of social policy pertaining to children in the UK as the development of child welfare law frequently mirrors changing social attitudes. Ideologies concerning child care in this country can be contradictory. When families function without criticism children are regarded as a private responsibility and motherhood is defined as a personal choice, but when families are considered dysfunctional the state will intervene on the basis that children are a public responsibility.

The current preferred state provision for children who cannot live with their own families is to place them with substitute/foster families, generally to be looked after by a female carer. Child-care norms, corresponding to national statistics, are that most children's primary carer is the mother so this would appear to confirm that the state's general choice meets societal expectations. However, in order that she can be available for this purpose most women need to be dependent upon a wage-earning partner, and it could thus be argued that child welfare policies which support this arrangement are entrenched in pre-existing beliefs and structures of female caring, part of which are women dependent upon male partners in 'traditional' families.

Since the 1970s there has been much political rhetoric about 'supporting the family', though past underfunding in public expenditure for expectations regarding health, social security and welfare have failed to keep up with demand. Partly as a consequence and in order to fill this gap, the principle that women are their families' carers has become enshrined in community care and the development of social work. This has underpinned arguments that, in the past, social policies have upheld particular values, normally in favour of men, and thus maintained major inequalities between the sexes.

Although at a macro level an analysis of state policies demonstrates that they do maintain and reinforce traditional patterns of gender beliefs, this may be an unintended consequence. It is easier for men to present 'legitimate excuses' as to why they are not able to provide care for others. Nevertheless, in effect, state social policies operate within a set of assumptions that are gender biased with the result that, usually, women act as unpaid carers within the home. There is thus a substantial literature that argues that state policies assume and prescribe a traditional nuclear family in which women are the main carers and that there are assumptions about the nuclear family as the preferred norm.

The family, however, is continuously being shaped by wider, outside structural forces so that modifications in family life cannot be separated either from other social changes, or from shifts within the sphere of intimacy. Daily life is consequently closely related to politics whilst policy also occurs in micro settings. Families do not react only to structural changes or to state policy; family members also have their own agency.

But how much agency do individual foster carers enjoy? Their daily life is prescribed by statute, by bureaucracy and by the custom and practice of social services departments. They have felt the demanding effect of the practice guidelines of the 1989 Children Act. Based on a series of research projects, the Act is couched in terms of a service to the children's birth families, not to the needs of foster carers' domestic lives, and was derived from the concerns of professional child welfare specialists. Its three main principles (the wishes of the child, non-intervention and joint parenting) have all ensured that the foster carer's task has become increasingly testing. Foster carer life has been further challenged by diminishing residential alternatives for the most difficult children, together with decreasing local authority budgets. As a result there are more troubled children under more adverse circumstances needing to be looked after in foster families and, in effect, this means by female carers. Ideologies concerning women and caring are so entrenched that they can lead to taken-for-granted assumptions: systems may thus depend upon socially invisible female work. A foster 'system of care' depends upon the work of women within the private domain, and this chapter seeks to discover how visible, or invisible, is the work of foster carers.

The history of foster care can be traced to biblical references to children cared for by unrelated adults. Historians also posit that growing up in another (foster) family may have been common early in the first millennium. There is evidence that, not infrequently, Viking children were raised in more noble families whilst medieval parents, where appropriate, arranged for their sons to be brought up in a family of the guild to which they were apprenticed. Colton (1998) refers to both abandoned children, and those of the affluent, being cared for by wet nurses during the Middle Ages in France, whilst English sixteenth-century records note that young orphans were placed with nurses. The formal boarding out of poor children in England, however, was first legalised by Hanway's Act of 1767.[1] This was later overtaken by, primarily Victorian, institutional provision which organised basic physical care for destitute children in line with the 1834 Poor Law's prevailing principles concerning the care of needy children.

A Report of a Drawing-room Conference on Boarding-Out Pauper Children (1876) documents the inception of the institutional form of foster care. 'Deserving' children might be rescued from the Work House to be boarded out with private families. The report indicates that fostering was a means of cutting the (escalating) cost of poor relief and a means of instilling the 'right' values in children by, for example, preparing them for work. This primary source gives the origins of the state foster care system, revealing that, in many ways, the issues remain the same. Gradually, during the nineteenth century, fostering came to be regarded as a charitable act; a means of rescuing children and placing them with substitute families with no thought of reunification. It was considered a long-term commitment and the use of the word foster 'parent' indicates the surrogate nature of the role. Parker (1990) refers to a 'child saving movement' and traces the history of foster care through the nineteenth century as a response to dual needs: a belief that, although male children could fend for themselves within the Work House, young girls should be protected from this, together with a perceived middle-class need for better-trained female domestics. Interest in the scheme accelerated when, in the twentieth century, it became clear that fostering was cheaper than the upkeep of institutions.

During the Second World War, large-scale evacuation of children brought to national attention both an increased public awareness of their needs together with an official concern for those without a 'normal' home life. The death of Dennis O'Neill in 1945 from neglect and abuse by his foster parents led to the Curtis Committee official inquiry which exposed the low standard of foster care supervision by unqualified Poor Law Officers. Its 1946 report recommendations laid the foundations for a professional child-care service and argued in favour of fostering as the best form of substitute care since the children 'bore a different stamp of developing personality and despite occasional misfits were manifestly more independent' (Curtis Report, 1946).

This was supported by the Home Office, then responsible for child care, because 'boarding out is the least expensive method both in money and in manpower and . . . it is imperative to exercise the strictest economy consistent with a proper regard for the interests of the children' (Home Office, cited by Bebbington and Miles, 1990: 284).

The 1948 Children Act acknowledged the importance of fostering as a child-care resource, set up the new Children's Departments and shifted the balance to recognise that children could be returned to their families. Bowlby's *Child Care and the Growth of Love*, published in 1953, lent further support for fostering (rather than residential care) when he identified the importance of meeting children's emotional needs via an exclusive maternal bond. Consequently, not only were increasing numbers of children placed in foster families in times of crisis but fostering became regarded as a 'natural' activity for women, and one that required little or no special training. As a result the culture of many foster families was to continue to offer substitute, rather than complementary, parenting with no regard for the children's birth families.

The Seebohm Report (Great Britain: Committee and Allied Personal Social Services, 1968) recommended the amalgamation of three local authority departments, Mental Health, Welfare and Children, into one social service department. Against the gains was a child-care loss with the dispersion of the expertise which for 20 years had supervised children in foster families.

Thus, mainly for financial reasons, the underlying principles of foster care have become care in the community rather than in an institution, together with a bid to give children the ordinary 'normal' family life it is presumed to provide (Packman, 1993). Homes which, in the perceptions of those organising the placements, most closely conformed to what Packman refers to as their 'bourgeois ideal', giving preference to a working father and a fully available mother. This is a stereotype which, as Sinclair and colleagues (2004) note, survives as current foster care households continue to reflect the selectors' conservative standpoint.

During the 1970s fostering was predominantly for young children whilst adolescents were cared for in children's homes. However, a crisis of confidence in residential provision during the 1980s, caused by low morale and the detection of instances of institutional maltreatment, resulted in government pressure to increase the supply of foster families, particularly as a cheaper alternative. This was a policy encouraged by the Audit Commission who recorded that 'the potential for improving value for money by increasing the percentage of children placed with foster parents continues to exist'[2] (1985: 2). This, together with a fundamental child-care tenet that every child has a right to 'normal family life', meant that fostering became part of institutionalised welfare.

Successive child-care policies and their underpinning legislation were rethought with the Children Act, 1989. This had a marked effect upon foster care. The Act's overarching principles are the paramountcy of the welfare of the child, the duty of public authorities to support families and children, a preference for negotiated solutions rather than court orders and the concept of enduring parental responsibility. The term 'parental rights' was replaced by 'parental responsibilities' which remain even when children live elsewhere, for example with a foster family. Thus, in many cases, the foster carer becomes pivotal as s/he may have to actively consult and negotiate with parents about decisions affecting the child. The duty of the foster carer is that s/he should:

> care for the child as if he [sic] were a member of the foster parents' [sic] own family, and . . . promote his welfare having regard to the local authority's long and short term arrangements for the child.
>
> (Department of Health, 1991: 140)

Shaw and Hipgrave (1989a) document the change of nomenclature from foster 'parent' to foster 'carer'. Since the mid-1970s the UK has witnessed the development of specialist fostering initiatives and they suggest that this name-shift was in recognition of carers' skills and expertise. Yet there remains some ambivalence in official documents which continue to refer to foster 'parents'.[3] The Fostering Network (NFCA, 1987a) recommends foster 'carers' in order to underline the difference for the child and to reinforce the continuing role of birth parents. This indistinctness in government terminology is indicative of a much wider ambiguity regarding the foster carers, which will be discussed in later chapters.

The original nineteenth-century assumption that divorcing children from their origins was the great panacea has changed. It is now considered that many of these children have problems even after their 'rescue'. They are seen, not as 'children without families', but as 'children from families with problems'. Social work belief is that effective work with children should take into account their origins, family networks and cultural environments, a notion generated by ecological theory, and that the child placed away is a product or 'symptom' of a dysfunctional interaction between the family and its environment. Thus any help should involve the whole family. Foster carers are centrally placed for the aspirations of this ecological perspective. In theory they are no longer substitute parents but more an extension of family support. The definition of a 'child of the family' in the Children Act excludes a child living with foster carers, thus reinforcing the view of fostering as a temporary arrangement. Yet, at the same time, the foster carer is responsible for all the common experiences associated with children's lives: peer relationships, opportunities for school achievement, community activities and an 'ordinary family setting'. Foster care is about providing a 'normal' life.

Local authority child welfare services provide a continuum of family placement from short-term fostering through to long-term permanency and on to adoption. In a bid to include all foster carers, Colton and Williams' discussion of an international description produces a 'somewhat clumsy working definition'. They suggest:

> 'Foster care' is care provided in the carers' home, on a temporary or permanent basis, through the mediation of a recognised authority, by specific carers, who may be relatives or not, to a child who may or may not be officially resident with the foster carers.
>
> (1997: 48)

Foster carers can either be friends, extended family or stranger carers to the child. The 1989 Children Act encourages the use of family and friends before those recruited by the local authority.[4] Families who care for kin children cannot expect financial help as a right. Rhodes posits that the resources offered to kin carers are restricted in order to uphold the notion of kinship obligation and family responsibility. As she comments: 'Foster care exposes . . . contradictory expectations at their starkest' (Rhodes, 1995: 182). Stranger foster carers are at least reimbursed a set amount for the child's expenses.[5]

In England anyone can apply to be a foster carer, although they must undergo a rigorous assessment process before being approved. Once registered with their local authority, all foster carers, including those working with an IFP, are then expected to work 'in partnership' with social services staff in order to care for the child(ren) placed with them. Although the term 'partnership' is not found in the legislation it is laid out in the 1989 Children Act Guidance, though an official comment notes, 'Arrangements between carers and authorities would be improved if foster carers are treated as full partners' (Utting, 1997: 28).

In order to understand the part that foster carers play it is important to consider the organisational and institutional setting within which foster care is delivered. Children placed by social services departments with registered foster carers are children in state care. In Britain the local authorities have some freedom to define policy and to fix budgets as they deliver most services, so there is considerable variability in both the structure of foster care services and its terminology. In addition, different parts of the United Kingdom have their own history of welfare and their own legislative systems so that there are differences between the component countries.

Alongside these differences the focus of the social workers' concerns has modified from decade to decade. In the 1960s there was an emphasis on preventing reception into care which, after a series of scandals, changed during the 1970s. Public condemnation following the death of Maria Colwell at the hands of her stepfather, after she had been removed by the court from a relative foster placement, resulted in an increase in the numbers of children removed from their families.

There is evidence that the characteristics of the children in foster care have become progressively more challenging over the years. Early adversity frequently results in difficult behaviours. 'They might steal, break things, have tantrums, refuse to eat, smear walls, wet their beds, refuse to bath, continually defy their carers, set light to their bedding, take overdoses, make sexual advances to other children, expose themselves in public, make false allegations, attack others, truant, take drugs or get into trouble with the police' (Sinclair *et al.*, 2004: 4). The 1975 Children Act produced another shift within the care system: a belief in psychological parenting resulting in the concept of 'professional' or 'specialist' fostering and expectations of 'treatment' for the children. The aim of specialist schemes was to ensure that children would not just be 'looked after' but that an additional ingredient would in some way ameliorate their characters and their attitudes.

Shaw and Hipgrave's survey (1983) of specialist foster care schemes revealed that social services were not offering the carers any career, pay or support services and that foster care had become the dumping ground for inappropriate and unplanned placements. Rushton's review (1989) confirmed that foster carers received little support. He describes them as exploited, treated insensitively with inadequate help and in need of a counselling service to manage rejection from children. There was little or no training on safer caring[6] or on how to handle disclosure of abuse. He also underlines the need to determine the status of foster carers within social service departments. This is confirmed by Sellick (1994) who found that foster carers' most frequent complaints related to the social workers, both with regard to the children and to themselves. He concludes that successful fostering depends upon good rapport between the parties and observes the need for praise and reassurance since the local authority expects so much accountability in return. Even today there is always a presumption that foster carers are available, often at short notice, to take in children and attend meetings or court. It is assumed that they will accept a multitude of additional tasks, for example the assessment of children, contact with the birth families in the foster home, supporting the family whilst the child is with them and often assisting young people after they leave. Yet Colton (1998) comments that many foster carers are still treated, by social services staff, as service recipients rather than as service providers.

In order to assist carers, local authorities now provide Family Placement social workers who, in their support of the placement, proffer help, advice and training to the foster carers. Triseliotis and colleagues' study of fostering in Scotland (1998) confirms earlier findings of general satisfaction with this part of the social care department. The *UK National Standards for Foster Care* (NFCA, 1999) recommend that these workers are called Supervising Social Workers in order to underline the growing expertise of the foster care service as it moves away from a body of well-meaning and untrained volunteers/foster carers to more specialist schemes supported by dedicated, trained personnel. As with many of the caring organisations, a contemporary trend in foster care has been its own professionalisation. Foster carers, as well as demonstrating the individual concern of a parent, have also to behave as though foster children are a professional responsibility; 'looking after someone else's child as though s/he is your own' (DHSS, 1955: 14) is no longer enough. As noted, most foster children have considerable needs and display challenging behaviours; their carers must work alongside staff from the courts, special education and health. In his Appendix A, Sellick (1992) lists some 30 skilled tasks that carers need to perform adequately since fostering encompasses children with many different needs; foster carers have to be 'parents plus'.[7] A report looking at the education of children within the looked-after system lists 14 complex tasks expected of foster carers (SSI/OFSTED, 1995), for example assessing the child's developmental needs across a range of circumstances. Although local authority specialist schemes include a fee-paying element, the majority of foster carers are not paid to do these multifarious tasks.

The Fostering Network lists ten statements of good practice with its seventh being: 'professional status for foster carers – as the equal partners of other professionals in the fostering team, receiving the full cost for a child plus payment for their skills and experience' (NFCA, 1987b). But foster carers are not credited with professional recognition by those who appoint them, and a series of critical reports in the 1990s suggests that councils' social care departments marginalize the service. Serious failings were identified by the Social Services Inspectorate (1996) in their report of six authorities. A 1997 report by the Association of Directors of Social Services (ADSS) was equally critical, exposing some complacency and identifying that although two-thirds of looked-after children were in foster care, yet greater attention and priority was still given to residential provision. Concurrently, Waterhouse's study (1997) on the organisation of the foster care services, gathered from data of 88 per cent of the local authorities in England, confirms considerable variation in the management and resultant quality of the foster care service. Intrinsic within these three reports is a view of the foster care service as undervalued and forgotten. In 1998 the government launched their 'Quality Protects' campaign, making available funds to improve the management and delivery of services for children. Money was, for example, provided for the recruitment, retention and training of foster carers.

A large-scale study in Scotland (Triseliotis *et al.*, 2000) describes a fairly optimistic foster care service with nonetheless persistent difficulties concerning the children's social workers, finance and general lack of support and consultation. These findings are mirrored in three further linked surveys of foster carers in seven local authorities over six years (Sinclair, Gibbs and Wilson, 2004; Sinclair, Wilson and Gibbs, 2000). They observe that one-third of study carers who had fostered for less than one year, and two-thirds of the whole sample, had experienced an incident which had a significant negative impact upon their family. Triseliotis and colleagues (2000) argue that the foster carers' status within social services remains ambiguous; they are neither colleagues nor service users and, behind the local authority rhetoric, there are few examples of working in partnership. Many foster carers describe the reality of their lives in terms close to the experiences Waterhouse recounted:

> foster carers perceived themselves as having low status and little information or influence; many respondents did not perceive themselves as part of an active team working together with social workers and parents to find a satisfactory outcome for a child.
>
> (1992: 43)

This lack of information is apparently mutual. The 1996 SSI report identifies a general lack of knowledge and experience concerning foster care amongst council staff. Schofield and colleagues (2000) confirmed this, noting that social workers are reluctant to advise foster carers and feel incompetent about giving guidance on the management of children's behaviour. A conference report (NCB/DoH, 2003) records that, although nationally foster carers felt that their status was improving, there remains lack of clarity about their role and what they do. Their work is unseen, hidden from scrutiny, so it is difficult to measure the quality of their care or their activities.

The four principles of fostering are localisation (close proximity to home and social networks), voluntariness (agreement rather than compulsion/court order), normalisation (the experience of family and the community) and participation (the involvement of child, birth parents, local authority and foster carers in the aims of the placement). Research has consistently shown that fostering is principally a temporary/short-term service for younger children, but alongside this there is a range of local authority care including respite (often for children with disabilities), 'specialist' schemes (for example, for youngsters remanded by courts), pre-adoption placements and assessment placements to aid determination of the child's long-term needs. In addition some foster carers offer children permanency, the continuity of relationships with caretakers and a family for life. Waterhouse (1997) observes that there are 47 terms for different fostering categories determined by the length of time, characteristic of the child (e.g. sibling group), or style/purpose of the placement (e.g. mother and baby assessment). Generally, many foster carers look after children with highly complex needs.

But what is known about these 37,000 families that foster? Although they are crucial to both the concept and to the service they have not commanded nearly as much research as the young people they look after. Yet the 1997 ADSS report states:

Nevertheless, without fully understanding why and how it works, the majority of us will say that foster care service is the favoured choice when seeking placements for children needing our care. It is of note that there is an absence of any large scale definitive research about the effectiveness of foster care in relation to other forms of looked after services. We as professionals still clearly *believe*[8] it is.

(1997: 4)

Is there research evidence for this belief? Comparative studies of the care provided for children in 12 residential homes with that provided by 19 foster families suggests that the interpersonal interactions are qualitatively different (Colton, 1988). Whilst staff in the residential sector monitor and supervise the children, foster carers continuously and personally relate with them. The children's attitudes, activities and emotional states matter as foster carers take an individual interest in, and concern for, their performance and well-being.

Research interest in foster carers has been mainly concerned with their selection, assessment and retention in order to inform future recruitment (for example, Adamson 1973; Gray and Parr, 1957). Recent large-scale studies, including the work of Rowe and colleagues (1984), Triseliotis' review (1989), Bebbington and Miles' surveys (1990), Triseliotis and colleagues' study of Scottish fosterers (2000) and the extensive work of Sinclair *et al.* (2004), offer more facts concerning foster carers. Foster carer profiles are found to be similar to that of the national pattern of adults except that they are older than parents of similar-aged children in the general population, with slightly more being house owners. Triseliotis and colleagues (1998) note some differences: 80 per cent own a car and 60 per cent of the households include at least one carer who smokes. His findings confirm previous studies with regard to active membership of religious groups. There is general confirmation of findings with regard to carers' close links to the caring professions and to the foster family form, typically traditionally nuclear.

Most studies concentrate upon the female carer with scant regard for the relevance of male carers.[9] Shaw and Hipgrave's survey (1989a) reveals that the selection of foster carers is becoming more liberal, including single people of both sexes. Wheal (1999a) establishes that 25 per cent of carers are single parents, though gives no gender breakdown. Sinclair and colleagues report (2000) that 24 per cent of their surveyed carers describe themselves as lone parents, with 55 per cent of these from ethnic minorities.

Further information can be culled from research that focuses on the characteristics of 'successful' foster carers. 'Success' in this instance being measured by the outcomes for the children rather than for the carers and, therefore, assessed against breakdowns in placement, or where researchers consider that the child has 'benefited' or 'been helped', rather than seek any alternative definition from the foster carers themselves. Positive factors attributed to 'successful' fostering include a willingness to work in an inclusive way (both with the child's birth family and the department), a disparity in the ages of the foster carers' own children vis-à-vis the fostered children, the importance of ongoing training, and the need for clarity with regard to expectations and role (Triseliotis, 1989). Thoburn (1995) adds to this a positive enjoyment of the company of children, flexibility, non-judgemental attitudes and an ability to negotiate. Later work (Sellick and Thoburn, 1997) identifies people who do not see the child as seriously problematic and so respond positively to challenging and difficult behaviour whilst expecting nothing back from the children. Sinclair and colleagues (2000) confirm 'successful' placements to be dependent upon carers who are seen by social workers as warm, encouraging and committed, with 'stickability'. Most research identifies that foster carers believe that they have something to offer needy children. But Colton and Williams (1998) review the several studies on characteristics of successful foster carers and conclude that they are inconclusive and contradictory.

Much of the research reviewed so far is from studies focusing on the children with information from social services staff plus postal surveys of foster carers. The carers are not the main focus but regarded as peripheral to the children and to the foster care system. A publication on foster care in general (Wheal, 1999b) does not actually contain a section specifically on them. As Sellick and colleagues observe (2004), research has generally considered foster carers only in terms of biography (marital status, family size, age and ethnicity), personality characteristics, motivation and values. Yet foster care is described as 'the fundamental bedrock on which we build our looked after children services' (Wheal, 1999b: 3). So how do foster carers provide this 'bedrock'? How do they manage the complexities of caring for a 'mix' of children – birth, fostered and possibly adopted? What is their experience of looking after some children for 'free' whilst replicating the same tasks for others involves an allowance or even a fee? Is there any literature which relates the foster carers' own perceptions and gives their world view? Where are the voices of the foster carers themselves? This next part of the review considers some of the literature which listens to these.

There are few studies where, not only are the foster carers used as primary sources, but they are also seen as people in their own right. Gray and Parr (1957) interviewed 438 'recruited' foster mothers using a pre-scripted questionnaire. Responses included that a child brings happiness into a home and that fostering itself is worthwhile. But there were fears regarding both how the children would 'turn out' and that, once fond of the child, the birth parent could remove. There was discontent over financial arrangements. Jenkins' study of 97 foster homes (1965), also for recruitment purposes, found that fostering fulfils compelling and unconscious needs. Foster carer motivations included feelings of loss, a need to compensate for their own poor parenting, a desire for (more) children and some compassion for children in need.

Adamson described her interviews of foster mothers 'as an attempt to get a sociological picture of the foster family' (1973: 103). The women were asked how they perceived themselves and their role; whether they liked thinking of themselves as a foster mother. The study revealed that whilst they might have a clear understanding of what the role of foster mother meant, 57 per cent of them rejected the role; they wanted to be the fostered child's 'actual' mother.

Foster Care: A Guide to Practice (DHSS, 1976) is based on written submissions from fostered children, foster care groups and individual foster parents. The result is a miscellany of practice wisdom and research findings. The foster carers consider their task hard work but worthwhile. They are aware that the general public is ambivalent about their role, viewing them as helpful and sentimental whilst simultaneously criticising them for putting their own children at risk from the effects of fostering. Some of this is replicated in interviews of American foster mothers (Hampson and Tavormina, 1980) which focus on their motives, rewards, regrets, specific problems and styles of discipline. The study concludes that carers' difficulties with the foster children are exacerbated by their own lack of legal rights and uncertainty about the children's lengths of stay. The women are critical of the number of moves foster children experience and aware of the resulting detrimental effect. As foster mothers they have no control over this yet feel blamed by the social care services. The authors note that 'the general ineffectiveness of foster care is placed upon the foster parent' (p. 108). Interestingly the thesis of a concurrent British study (Edwards, 1980) is that the stresses of foster care are too great to be managed by the professional support services. This dilemma of responsibility is observed by Jassal (1981) in his study of short-term carers, most of whom perceive themselves as substitute parents to the children. The great majority – 80 per cent – experience fostering as both more difficult and more rewarding than anticipated. He argues that in all cases it fills a need in the carers' lives so that it is as important to the foster carer as to the child that the placement should succeed. Because of the intensity of daily care, carers become very attached to the children; 90 per cent of the families find letting the children go difficult and painful. Foster carers' high commitment was also identified by Rowe and colleagues' (1984) interviews of 39 foster carers (focusing on 'success') and conversely a study reflecting the experiences of 11 foster families where placements had ended prematurely (Aldgate and Hawley, 1986).

Research to elucidate any characteristics which would aid the identification of 'really excellent long term foster parents, as distinct from parents who were just adequate' (Dando and Minty, 1987: 387) sought information from foster mothers and social services staff. The researchers listened to the views of 80 foster mothers on the impact of fostering on family life. The decision as to which of the foster mothers were adequate and which were excellent was a judgement made by the social workers who rated the carers' overall performance according to three criteria: agency-role understanding, basic child care and special capacities. The study concludes that the motives most closely associated with excellent fostering are childlessness, a general social conscience and an identification with deprivation based on personal experience. The benefits of fostering seemed closely related to motivation, particularly for the childless foster mothers who found satisfaction in nurturing children. Generally the study found that high standards of fostering were associated with drives based on, or derived from, strong personal needs. It established that foster mothers who gave as their primary motive 'liking children' were not highly rated. Although the study does not tell us how the foster mothers evaluated their own experience and their own performance, it gives us insights into what they considered to be their compensations.

Berridge and Cleaver's more ambitious survey of 372 placements (1987) also sought the views of the foster carers on specific issues. One of their findings concerns the unequal power dimension between the carers and the social workers, to the perceived detriment of the carers. The authors query whether this may, in fact, serve organisational interests. Their research includes ten in-depth phenomenological case studies. For each of these they sought to interview some eight people (e.g. child, social worker, teacher) including the foster carers. It is worthy of note that, in their methodology, they give numbers for all categories except for the carers. When the same list is repeated later in the study the authors do not mention the foster carers. It takes some searching to discover that all the carers agreed to be interviewed. This actually mirrors their own findings: that files were kept on less than 25 per cent of the carers and that, of those in existence, half held virtually no information and all were kept with the clients' files. Like the local authorities, the researchers render the carers invisible.

The role of payment for caring is examined by Leat (1990) through interviews of four different groups of carers, including foster carers. The other groups were remunerated but foster carers were in receipt of allowances only, paid fortnightly in arrears. Although dismissive of the 'costs' of caring they talked of its manifold stresses, the isolation, the children's destructive and antisocial behaviour and their lack of recognition. Nonetheless they felt that they were involved in worthwhile tasks as they perceived the children as being in considerable need and derived satisfaction from them, despite their behaviour. A similar ambivalence pervades a study concerning contact with birth families (Waterhouse, 1992). Her examination of the perceptions, attitudes and experiences of 17 short-term carers demonstrates the complexity and ambiguity of their situation. Cleaver's (2000) research explores the impact of contact on all concerned (foster carers, birth family, foster children) without giving any of the participants particular weighting. Foster carers found it problematic but were more likely to promote contact if trained and well supported.

A study interviewing foster carers and considering support/training concludes that the importance of foster care is its intangible rewards (Butler and Charles, 1999). Foster carers have an expectation of reciprocity of emotional attachment and gratitude; of children so wanting to become part of the family that they, themselves, will change in order to 'fit in'. Drawing upon a particular theoretical framework the researchers suggest that the effects of not getting these rewards leads to a deterioration in the carers' role satisfaction. It means that they focus on the hurts, or blame the social services department. The tangible rewards (payment and training) are insufficient as compensation. Butler and Charles do not quote directly from the foster carers but mediate their experiences, perceptions and opinions within their own conceptual paradigm.

An analysis of 918 foster carers' survey returns (Triseliotis *et al.*, 2000) is checked against further qualitative material obtained from interviews of 67 carers. These interviews were open-ended but centre on specific key issues and demonstrate that many carers feel overloaded by difficult children and increased demands and hence perceive themselves as frequently ill supported. Yet, although the majority find fostering hard, they also find it rewarding. The three main motivations for fostering emerge as 'having something to offer', a fondness for children with an awareness of 'need' coupled with 'wanting to put something back' into the community. The benefits and attractions of fostering centre jointly around the progress that the children make, a sense of achievement and job satisfaction (70 per cent) whilst the other 30 per cent say that it enhances their lives, makes them feel that they are doing something worthwhile and gives them an insight into the problems of others. Schofield and colleagues' interviews of 43 foster carers (2000) identify three categories: 'family builders', 'second families' and 'professionals'. Most feel that parenting is what they do best, are motivated by altruism and positively enjoyed the 'bustle' of family life but have to negotiate between being a real family for the foster child and being foster carers for the local authority.

Overall this brief review offers us glimpses into foster carers' worlds but the information is frequently closely framed by the research question of each study. Warren (1999) suggests that this shortage of in-depth studies of foster care, compared to that of residential care, reflects the low priority and status accorded to the service and, one might add, to the place of the foster carer.

This chapter has outlined the history and development of foster care. It has summarised the social research literature with particular emphasis on the foster carers themselves. It has sought, but not found, much prominence given to their perspectives. For foster carers altruism provides motivation (Schofield *et al.*, 2000; Triseliotis *et al.*, 1998), whilst allowances mean that they can remain home-based (Rhodes, 1993). There are indications that they are marginalised: some poor communication with local authorities (Sellick, 1994), treated as service recipients rather than colleagues (Colton, 1989) and problems with social workers (Triseliotis *et al.*, 2000). Fostering can damage family life (Sinclair *et al.*, 2004). Foster carers describe fostering as difficult but rewarding (Jassal, 1981) because children bring happiness (Gray and Parr, 1957) and many carers want to be their 'real' mothers (Jenkins, 1965) in order to increase the size of their families (Dando and Minty, 1987; Rowe *et al.*, 1984).

Much of the information on foster carers comes either from large-scale questionnaires and surveys, or from a social service focus relying upon the opinions of the social workers to assess the criteria for successful outcomes for foster children. But social care departments and foster carers have different frames of reference. Perhaps it is because the views and perceptions of social services staff are so dominant that those of the foster carers have often been overlooked and neglected. It seems that foster carers have no narrative rights and, as a result, it is possible to piece together only a fragmented and incomplete picture. Foster carers are seen as tangential to the foster children.

The review indicates that the social research theoretical base for foster care originates from a local authority belief that foster carers should demonstrate heightened parenting skills (much like adoptive parents and stepparents) for caring for other people's children. Yet the majority of children in public care pass through the foster care system so that the official role of the foster carer is to prepare the child for a return home, or a move on to another permanent family. Foster carers are now considered not as parents, but as carers. How do the carers themselves manage this change? The literature which hints at their perceptions, their world view or their explanations of how they understand their lives as foster carers is limited. As there is no body of academic work which is both substantially and empirically pertinent to foster carers, it is therefore necessary to seek the theoretical frameworks from elsewhere. It may be that an understanding of this will help to bring foster carers into sharper focus and transfer their voices from the perimeter into the centre.

2 Towards a theorising of foster care

A review of the social work and social research publications on foster care produces a body of material related to foster carers, but little that explores their world views. Any foster care literature focusing on the carers tends to cover only the practicalities of looking after other people's children; most local authorities, for example, produce a foster care handbook. In order to develop any hypothesis it is necessary to draw on frameworks from elsewhere, from the three related concepts of public and private domains, caring and finally family and household. This literature should contribute to a theoretical framework for the practice of foster care and thereby make foster carers themselves more visible.

The split between public and private is an established central organising theme in feminist thinking and provides some basic orientations. The concepts can be discussed in terms of institutions, of space, of resources and of ways of knowing. Frequently they are dichotomised in terms of political/ personal, instrumental/expressive and male/female. Although not an accurate depiction of reality, this terminology aids description and can provide organising categories for the study of foster carers' lives. As a conceptual framework, insights around public and private may help emancipate (foster) families from 'theoretical invisibility' (Weintraub, 1997: 32) since carers offer what would normally be ideologically constructed as their private lives, their homes and their intimates as a public service for the care of children who are not usually blood relatives.

The ideological division of home (the private domain) and work (the public domain) is often tracked back to the late eighteenth century. Although the focus was on paid production, and not an analysis of the domestic arena, the separation of home and work has been attached to the processes of industrialisation. Originally women combined care-giving with production but it has been argued that when the two domains became separate, men commandeered the public world of paid employment, leaving women the private world of home and intimacy (Waerness, 1989). From this emerged the idea of the household sphere as a private space for domesticity, though Rose (1986) warns against overstating this split. For many women the home continued to be an important site for wage earning and some foster carers may place themselves in this category (Moralee, 1999; Adamson, 1973).

Although the terms 'public' and 'private' are ideological distinctions rather than empirical categories, people nevertheless expect their public and private lives to make different claims and to offer different benefits. In daily life these distinctions are so continuously constructed that they operate as norms within society. Assumptions associated with this division are that the 'public domain' is male (paid work and authority, rationality, culture, politics and power), whilst that of the 'private domain' is female (hearth and home, emotion, children and domestic labour). The private is regarded as being of less authority and lower status, and structural oppression ensures that the position of women remains subordinate (Edwards, 1990). Private and public is thus about different domains, statuses, ways of behaving, ways of being (Edwards, 1993), and also different ways of caring.

'Professional' care, within the public domain, is described (theoretically) as rational, scientific and male in contrast to female care, in the private domain, which is perceived as natural, instinctive and emotive. Waerness (1987) suggests that the Welfare State, the public face of care, could learn from women's experience in the private sphere in order to restore qualities which have been lost in its professionalisation. A comparative study of children's homes and foster care concludes that the interpersonal inter-actions within the two are qualitatively different as Colton (1989) shows that foster carers have much to offer/teach residential staff. This is unlikely to occur because, as Waerness (1987) explains, it would threaten profes-sionals and undermine their bureaucratic control (rational care). In fact, in some local authorities it is the professional (salaried) staff in residential units who offer advice to (unpaid) foster carers. The dominant, rational care philosophy of the public social services is that their staff are considered the 'experts'.

Foster carers have to deal continuously with this reality of bureaucracy. Although the activities of mothers are increasingly the concern of public authorities (Brannen and O'Brien, 1995; Ribbens, 1994) in theory, the family is ideologically constructed as an area for non-intervention. But foster carers are subject to registration and regular inspection. Their care of other peoples' children is constantly monitored and constrained by social services staff; there are explicit instructions – for example, all babysitters must be police checked. A service provided within the private domain becomes public property. Foster carers thus actively demonstrate Saraceno's (1984) discussion concerning the interpenetrations and integrations between the two spheres of public and private, and the fragility and fluidity of their boundaries.

The site of foster care is therefore one of ambiguity and potential conflict. Initially grounded in the ideology of the family and the private, domestic domain, foster family lives daily feel the impact of the public world via state intervention. This is ably demonstrated by the terminology. Originally foster children were cared for by foster parents: a foster mother and a foster father. The choice of vocabulary underlines the surrogate role and directives emphasised caring for the children 'as if they were a member of the foster parents' own family' (CM 2184, 1988). Fostering was considered an extension of the mothering role requiring those 'natural' female virtues that are characteristic of the familial space, described by Rhodes (1994) as 'a domestic vocation'. But foster parents are now foster carers, nomenclature taken from the public world of care. Adults who are thus 'parents' to one child are 'carers' to another and must manage this ambiguity within the same setting. Parenthood frequently mirrors changes of values in society so events in the public world shape the nature of care-giving in the private world of the foster family. Foster 'carers' must remember that the children they give their hearts to are only transitory. But how do these issues get worked out in the detail of their everyday lives in relation to ideas about 'caring' and 'mothering'? Do female carers model themselves on traditional motherhood or professional carers?

Women who have paid work in the public sphere also have to labour, for love and not for money, in the private sphere. They find themselves between two contradictory value systems (Feree, 1985), one overseen by exchange values (where work is governed by instrumental market relations) and the other by use value (where work is personal and for the satisfaction of others). Moving between these two worlds involves different ways of managing; there are tensions between the two. Foster carers cannot move physically from one to the other, like the office worker, but must organise the two together, home as work place; their concern for the children and the process of caring, together with the demands of the local authority. Some have to cope simultaneously with their own and fostered children, but in different ways; there are, for example, regulations about sanctions for foster children. State departments are goal oriented and driven by a means/end rationality which may be alien to the individual care of the private domain. Foster carers must manage the domestic/institutional dialectics of privacy versus surveillance, informality versus regulation and personal versus professional within one site (Peace and Holland, 1998). Rhodes suggests that the transfer of child-care provision from residential homes to foster families has also transferred the institutional characteristics. The additional bureaucratic regulations are eroding its 'ordinary' nature:

> Although fostering is referred to as 'informal care', the intrusion of these regulatory activities increasingly draws it closer to the formal sphere and, in the process, damages the very qualities of family life which it seeks to promote.
>
> (1993: 11)

If the role of the foster carer becomes more operational it risks losing its vital social interaction and qualitative 'feel': concentration on formal performance distracts from the experiential care of children. Foster carers must somehow retain their privately based experiences along with their more publicly based forms of knowledge and understanding.

This paradoxical situation with its inevitable tensions is analysed in a study of providers of home-based day-care; an ambiguous phenomenon of waged mothering (Nelson, 1990a). The providers experienced complex relationships with the children as their strong bonds of attachment were controlled by the contractual arrangements. Like foster carers they had none of the privileges of motherhood and only limited authority and responsibility. Their use of the mothering model not only interfered with business boundaries but upset the children's mothers who, anxious not to be displaced, set limits (Nelson, 1989). Much of this maps onto foster care. The children are placed under a contractual agreement and carers may have to mediate with both bureaucracy and birth parents.

This overview of some aspects concerning notions of public and private is oversimplified but furthers our understanding of foster carers' lives. Foster carers are situated at the overlap and the penetrations of the public/ private domains and the use of these concepts will help to elucidate their particular world views. As ideological distinctions, ideas concerning public and private aid the explanation of key features of daily life, although it is important to underline that different people at different times experience them in different ways. Brittan and Maynard (1984) highlight that because ideologies are 'common sense' and 'obvious' they often appear universal, natural and inevitable and become embedded; they can be powerful tools in the social system. Reviewing some of the literature on the ideologies around concepts of public and private explains women's particular relationship with the (less powerful) private domain, which Edwards argues (1993) is unlikely to change because of female responsibilities rooted in childbearing and child rearing. In order to understand this further it is helpful to look at some of the literature around caring and the influence of gender constructs.

Caring is 'typically defined by feminist researchers as the unpaid work of kin within the private domain of family' (Graham 1991: 6). Ideologically the main site of caring in post-industrial Western societies is the family and the home, since tenderness and emotion are more permissible there than anywhere else (Stacey and Price, 1981). Tronto (1993) describes caring as both a practice and a disposition; it is a private labour defined as a work of love. A 'labour of love', and a daily grind, as the word caring melds both concepts (Graham, 1983). Care is based on responsibilities and relationships and is therefore considered a moral activity. Waerness defines caring as 'a concept encompassing that range of human experiences which have to do with feeling concern for and taking charge of the well-being of others' (1987: 210).

Caring has thus both practical and psychological implications; it is about activities and feelings. Foster carers have a duty of care for the children they look after, which may relate in a complex way to moral imperatives, and to whether they organise care differently for their own birth children compared to those that they formally 'look after'. For foster children, like their own, they take responsibility both for practical matters (e.g. health checks) and also for the children's psychological well-being (as far as this is possible). Much of this is laid down in fostering handbooks. However, much is not specified in writing so that the carers only know that their care has been found wanting when they are criticised by the local authority. Care is only visible when it is not done (Graham, 1982). It is as though social services departments expect their foster carers (particularly the female carers) to know instinctively what constitutes quality care. They demand that foster carers involve both the department and the child's birth family; care within an 'inclusive' culture (Holman, 1975). It has to be private care in public mode in order to include the (bureaucratically acceptable) qualities of motherhood.

Boulton (1983) reviews the literature that regards motherhood as important for establishing women's femininity, respectability and maturity but child care as a low-status occupation. Tronto (1993) agrees that a mother's tenderness gains her an equal and just place in society whereas caring has become devalued. Yet because the primary skills required in fostering are understood as those of innate, natural mothering, foster carers are regarded as subordinates (Oldfield, 1997). Meyer (1985) comments that their position, because they are 'pretend' mothers, is treated as lower than 'ordinary' mothers: an ambiguous situation where skilled carers are nonetheless defined as of low status. Leat's study (1990) identified lack of recognition of foster carers' skills but, in contrast, noted that there were compensations – for example when carers were congratulated at school for progress achieved, which is unlikely to occur with their own birth children! Graham found that for some single women caring was 'the medium through which (they) are accepted into and feel they belong in the social world' (1983: 30). Caring can define identity, and this may resonate for some foster carers.

Fisher and Tronto (1990) note that one of the identifying features of care-giving is that women are assigned this responsibility but with little authority. Foster carers are responsible for care-giving, that is care as a relationship in which care is both given and received. Care-giving requires time, material resources, knowledge and skill (ibid.). The social care departments are responsible for supporting the carers with the latter three. They are charged to provide equipment, information, training and supervision. But it is the department which holds all the formal power, retaining the authority to register and to de-register the carers, to place and to remove the children. Yet, in order to ensure that public children are looked after within families the department is, paradoxically, dependent upon foster carers.

A review of informal care-providers (Parker, G., 1990) shows that families do usually care for dependants; there is no abrogation of this obligation. Nevertheless this care task is normally not shared but the responsibility of one person. Cancian (1986) notes that a 'feminisation of love' has resulted in the belief that it is 'natural' for women to be carers.

Women become responsible for caring tasks at both an ideological and a material level (Ungerson, 1983) and caring becomes part of their socially constructed self-identity (Graham, 1983). Backett's study of parents (1978) and how they negotiate care tasks for their children shows that there are assumptions that not only should mothers take overall responsibility for their children's care, but that they should also be constantly available. Most of the literature assumes that care is, in reality, gendered, a view challenged by Arber and Gilbert (1989). Their analysis of the 1980 General Household Survey shows that elderly men make a larger contribution than has been recognised to support disabled wives. They acknowledge, however, that there is a general expectation that married daughters should also help and, in overall terms, women still comprise the majority of carers (Abel and Nelson, 1990). Age Concern notes that one in five women are 'sandwich carers', responsible for both children and elderly parents (News in Brief, 1998).

Because of this cultural designation as carers, women with dependants (child or adult) find imposed, and thus often feel, an ethical imperative to provide care. Their special relationship with the private domain entails notions of duty and responsibility, particularly to children, and they thus embody in themselves the moral order. It is assumed that they will give priority to caring and to fulfilling immediate family needs. They become, ideologically speaking, the incarnate, moral and emotional centre of the home. Women are thus likely to get trapped into commitments and exchanges of support. Their identities as carers get constructed, confirmed and reconstructed (Finch and Mason, 1993).

'Good' caring is arguably concerned with the independence and autonomy of the cared for in order to encourage growth and development (Abel and Nelson, 1990). Foster carers are asked to prepare children for independence. Young people are frequently expected to leave foster families between the ages of 16 and 18 years and formal local authority support usually finishes by the age of 21. Thus, young people, whose early experiences mean that they often require more support and care, are expected to cope with independence some years before cultural expectations would consider them sufficiently able, and at a time when social policy is increasingly extending young adults' reliance on parental support (Jones and Bell, 2000). Lindsay (1994) notes that the average age that children in the care system 'leave home' is 16.5 years whilst for the general population it is 22.5 years. Many in this latter group have the option to return home in times of crisis and Jones (1995) argues that, because this option is used increasingly, leaving home is a process rather than an event. Nonetheless for those who have been fostered and have experienced the care of the private domain, their life course is dominated by the public domain's institutional care. The dilemma for foster carers is that even when they know intimately the difficulties of these youngsters, they may have to refuse further help, and to no longer care.[1]

Fisher (1990) traces the growth of female employment in the caring services from the need of single women to establish and define themselves as independent both of the household and of a husband. She extends her study to contemporary women's motivations for care work and identifies three interconnecting explanations: they recognise an unmet need, or feel themselves to be on a social mission, or personally wish to effect social change. Her argument is that capitalist and patriarchal structures favour male earners and thus limit and restrict women's choices. This context may indicate similar reasons for women's fostering. Adamson's study (1973) revealed very different motivations for foster mothers in economically disadvantaged areas (no waged alternative) than in more affluent regions (a wish to offer something to children). A finding confirmed both by Boulton (1983) with regard to the satisfactions of motherhood, and Moralee (1999) who linked foster carer availability to areas where employment opportunities were poor. Tronto (1993) explores the reasons for the devaluing of care; because care is associated with emotion, the needy and historically with servants and slaves, care is conceptually diminished and equated with weakness. It is a vicious circle; care is devalued and those people so engaged are deprecated. Both Berridge (1997) and Sellick (1992) refer to the low status ascribed to foster carers within the social services and attribute this to the fact that, as substitute parents, their work does not appear to require special skills. Although, because they are a scarce resource, carers are not always entirely powerless (Masson *et al.*, 1999). Tronto (1993) notes that where men become involved care work gains status and prestige as in, for example, the position of head waiter in an exclusive restaurant.

Many men are carers; recent large-scale surveys confirm that the majority of foster carers live as a couple (Sinclair *et al.* (2004), 63 per cent of 1416; Triseliotis *et al.* (2000), 78 per cent of 835). Nationally the local authorities' assessment and preparation of newly recruited foster carers involves both adults. Nonetheless there is an assumption that, once registered, it is the female carer who will take the lead role (Newstone, 1999). Much of the research reviewed in chapter 1 concentrated only on the views of female carers. There is scant information on male carers. It seems that there is little public expectation that male foster carers should be closely involved with the care of the children. Many studies in fact confirm that, whatever the rhetoric of 'new man', male participation in caring and domestic duties continues to lag.[2]

There are studies which focus on parents' and carers' responsibilities and world views in an effort to understand their perspectives. Boulton's (1983) study of mothers shows that although many considered the child a burden, nonetheless they derived great satisfaction from being needed. Nelson's (1990b) study of day-care providers made visible women who wanted to be loved and relied upon and actually invited the 'burden'. Whilst some felt that they were giving children the love that they themselves did not get, others could repay the love that they had received. All the providers believed that they treated the day-care children the same as their own. Because of this they felt that they drew most on their mothering skills. Even those that had professional care expertise, for example nursing qualifications, listed mothering before their training and their experience.[3] Thus it would seem that domestic caring is primarily defined by private ways of being, even when we might expect other orientations to be apparent. But what do foster carers draw upon for their care of other people's children? The first chapter noted the significant correlation between foster carers and their work experience, past and present, in the caring professions. As carers, do they use this expertise or do they draw on their parenting for the care of their fostered children?

Children in care are formally protected. Foster carers agree to certain conditions. Foster children may not be shouted or sworn at, or smacked; there are cautions regarding the physical expression of affection. There is thus a potential for conflict should carers wish/have to treat birth children and fostered children by different care standards. The Children Act, 1989, stipulates that fostered children have rights and that their wishes must be heard, although these are mediated by adults. Theoretically local authorities construct children as active, competent participants. But foster care has traditionally operated within a needs, not rights, framework and this risks competing interests between children and their carers. Children may not rely upon foster carers to represent their interests.

This discourse of rights places foster children within a public concept of justice. Ruddick (1996) reviews those arguments which root justice and care in different worlds. A morality of justice is part of the male, rational, separated world whereas a morality of care is part of the female, connected world, and particularly of the family. It could be argued that justice and care are philosophically incompatible, especially as care is particular (an individual foster child wants music lessons) and justice universal (all foster children receive pocket money). Ruddick extrapolates that in the same way that concepts of care are applied to the public sphere so should the language of justice, from the public domain, be applied to the family; they are not mutually exclusive. Tronto (1993) insists that a theory of care is not complete without justice. If foster children are protected by children's rights, does this mean that the conflict between care and justice maps onto conflicts between foster carers' birth children and foster children: does the concept of justice only apply to foster children? Rees (1996) describes how birth children negotiated increased pocket money in order to gain parity with the foster child.

Care versus justice provides a complex context as foster carers must continuously balance out differing needs. Nelson's (1994) day-care providers aimed to treat their own and other children with parity. Examination suggests that they discriminated against their own. Efforts to provide excellent mothering to the minded children affected their maternal role in relation to their birth children. Not only did they compromise their own standards of good mothering but they provided a service they disapproved of, since many of them childminded in order not to leave their own children for outside paid work. In a similar vein foster children are usually very needy whilst the carers' own children are comparatively stable. It is likely that foster carers' children will risk injustice as they experience an alteration in their own care.

Foster carers are caught between two different constructions of childhood: children as vulnerable and in need of protection, and children with rights. Ignatieff (1989) champions the cause of justice/rights demanding that welfare should be about this and not about caring, and wants citizenship built on entitlement, not altruism. He insists that, in a just society, care-receivers should not have to accept what care-givers decide they need. Rights entitle people to respect and dignity and no amount of care/charity is an adequate substitute. The Department for Education and Skills prescribes placement choice (rights) for foster children but too frequently they are cared for wherever there is a vacancy (Waterhouse, 1997).

Children are placed with foster families because of a belief that this is the optimum arrangement for their welfare. Fostered children also have their own birth families and the Children Act, 1989, insists that it is these families who are given priority. Wherever possible birth parents retain parental responsibilities, even when their children are cared for by a third party. It is the birth parents, not the foster carers, with whom the social services department must work in partnership. Birth families must be consulted and can give explicit instructions regarding their child, for example with regard to hair styles and menus. In day-care situations this undermines confidence and authority (Nelson, 1994). Foster carers are in a similar ambiguous position with regard to their relationships with the fostered children. They must juggle the competing needs of family members whilst maintaining a relationship with the foster child, frequently with the certainty of loss, and manage their own emotions concerning this.

It is arguably the emotional component in any relationship that makes it meaningful and fulfilling. Abel and Nelson (1990) posit that it is the emotional constituent that ensures that caring is not demeaning for either party. Caring relationships, however, do not always include affection; some rest on fear and obligation (Graham, 1983). Ungerson (1987) found that strong bonds can frustrate the delivery of care; in order to care for their elderly parents some daughters had to stop caring about them. Nelson's (1990a) day-care providers experienced difficulties if they became too attached; 77 per cent owned to emotional commitment. Most coped by 'detached attachment' and had to recreate this relationship daily with the children. Foster carers face similar emotional dilemmas; they love children, often to lose them, and cannot depend upon reciprocated affection in the interim.

Generally, within families mothers hold powerful positions, even if this may be circumscribed and contingent. They carry the knowledge of family life and can thus structure the contexts within which decisions get taken and organise the household to their own authoritative advantage (Ribbens, 1993a). But is this true of female foster carers who are no longer foster 'mothers'? Glenn (1994) questions whether shifts in language and imagery represent actual movement in thought, or simply the reconstitution of old ideas. Does this change of nomenclature invest the carers with more professionalism and therefore more power, or does it diminish their status to domestic carers?

Foster carers have an ambiguous parent/worker role with the children they look after. Of all the professionals concerned with the child they are the ones most vulnerable to becoming emotionally involved. It is the role of the carer to love and to lose (Jassal, 1981). Care involves both labour and love; Lynch's (1989) expression 'solidary labour' explains that labour and love cannot be analysed separately because of their reciprocal interdependence. Morgan (1996) suggests that there may be pressures in caring to shift to the more impersonal. A terminological 'shift' has occurred in foster care as foster mothers/fathers have now officially become foster carers, a more obscure and equivocal term which may affect the nature of the care relationship. Yet foster carers look after children within the privacy of their own homes, the site where expressions of emotion are not only permissible but expected. Household is the realm of particularistic ties.

Whilst Lynch (1989) argues that caring also occurs in several extra-familial contexts, other feminist writers place the locus of most caring within the informal privacy of home. Fostering occurs within the carer's household but is regulated by public authorities. There is a perceived need to monitor the care of the children to ensure minimum standards; there is an annual inspection of the child's bedroom. Foster carers have to work with the many state representatives who visit and check upon their care. They are obliged to explain their actions, countenance criticism, negotiate on behalf of the children, themselves and their own families. This is considered acceptable, expected accountability by the local authority 'experts' and 'professionals'. This claim to expertise by social workers gives them personal power.

Female foster carers mediate with a growing body of experts and professionals; they are becoming, as Graham (1985) describes, both 'providers and teachers'. Yet for all of this motherhood-writ-large, carers cannot insist upon being heard in relation to their foster children. It is not automatic that the 'experts' will request foster carers' views and opinions on the children that they care for daily. Foster carers have to entrust the futures of their foster children to the judgement of others. Foster carers have no rights (Lowe, 1994). The need for more collaborative working is recognised (Utting, 1997) but the research of Triseliotis and colleagues (2000) reveals that this is empty rhetoric. These tensions, inherent at the interface between foster carers and the social care personnel, are akin to those between mothers and teachers (Ribbens, 1993b). She questions how far mothers, who have responsibility for their children, also have authority; a dilemma possibly pertinent for foster carers.

Foster carers sign an undertaking to care for the child as if s/he were a member of their family. The belief is that 'family life' can offer additional qualities. Studies show that home day-care providers were certain that they offered something 'extra' compared to a day-care centre. They described this in emotional terms; that the centre did not proffer 'warmth, love and intimacy' (Nelson, 1994: 186). Comparative studies of the care provided in residential homes with foster families confirms these beliefs (Colton, 1988 and 1989). Whilst residential institutions 'cared for' the children, the foster families also 'cared about' them; the residential provision lacked an affective ingredient. The tangible performances of foster carers and residential staff were distinctly influenced by the contrasting actualities of home (personal, intimate, moral commitment) and the more bureaucratic institution (rule-governed where performance is motivated through financial incentives).

Formal state policy tends to reduce caring to work in the public sense: to rotas, shifts, statutory breaks and second-hand information so that it risks losing the 'love' dimension. Foster carers offer round-the-clock care and apply knowledge from intimate understandings, from particularistic ties, not abstract principles. Foster carers, as in Ruddick's theory of mothering (1983), learn through practice not instruction. The essence of care-giving is about attentiveness to detail. This is most efficacious within the context of an intimate relationship, between foster carer and foster child in the domestic/private domain, but foster carers' caring is heavily influenced by the social services. As a public sector body, social services is concerned not with detail but with a general set of rules. Thus the lives of foster carers epitomise a wider issue, that of how to legislate/bureaucratise family lives and particularistic ties.

Social services departments must ensure that children are 'cared for', that minimum standards concerning their health, education and general welfare are met. The preferred option is that children are placed with foster families. It is these families that 'care about' the children. These concepts identify distinctions which are not mutually exclusive. Caring and fostering children involves two rationalities (Ve, 1989). Foster carers need to identify themselves with the children in order to understand their individual requirements and adopt a caring, responsible rationality. The technical rationality of the local authority is primarily concerned with efficiency, economy and the maximisation of production. In practice the activity of parenting combines both aspects but at least mothers have some autonomy. Foster carers have to manage the conflicting aims of these two models of care and may experience the context for their care-giving as critical. It is the context which, if adverse, can impede them from fulfilling their idea of good care, particularly if there are constraints because of the bureaucratic structure and strictures of the social services departments.

Bureaucracies require routines and standardisation in order to operate; they deal with generalisations and not with detail. Thus if an individual's need is not standard then the care giver must rely on ingenuity to cope (Abel and Nelson, 1990). Foster carers, for example, regularly subsidise the children they look after (Oldfield, 1997); they meet those needs not yet recognised/formalised by the social services. Bureaucracy's need for standard techniques means that care becomes a component of the regulatory system: it is converted from a human service into a commodity. Foster carers have to work with this rationale which may become more problematic for those carers who, in receipt of a fee, may believe that they are paid to comply.

Care can be analysed in terms of whether it is paid or unpaid. There is much ideological support for the latter (underpinned by economic arguments), as witnessed by government initiatives for care in the community, which frequently means care by the community. Foster care could be described as one of the earliest examples of this. Historically foster care was conceived as an extension of parenting, rather than as work outside the domestic domain. Smith (1988) reasons that generally society believes that mothering is a skill which women owe humanity. This is explicit in some of the discussion which laid the foundations for British post-war child welfare: 'Although her labour deserves reward . . . the acceptance of payment for the work cuts at the root of the relation between foster mother and a child which we wish to create' (Curtis Report, 1946). A report of a London working party noted 40 years later, 'Extraordinarily, one local authority had reduced expenses to its foster parents on the basis that they should be "doing it for love"' (NFCA, 1986). Clearly payment and love may be seen as contradictory themes. Money is regarded as a visible symbol of service but there are also beliefs that 'money cannot buy love'. Issues regarding payment expose a key dilemma of the public/private debate regarding foster care. One of the beliefs in support of unpaid, 'for love' caring is that there is job satisfaction from emotional attachment. It is part of the ideological packaging of care with altruism and mothering. Studies of human services illustrate that people are drawn to certain occupations because of a desire to help (Abel and Nelson, 1990) and find that there are subjective rewards (Fisher, 1990). But are there different orientations for the task now that foster mothers have become foster carers and will this change these assumptions?

Cancian (1986) argues that the feminising of love and affective caring by society (dependent on an ideology that child care is for love, and is therefore not work) has contributed to the devaluation and exploitation of women. Oldfield (1997) argues that foster carers who view themselves as mothers are not concerned about payment. Smith (1988) shows that Australian foster carers demonstrate four sets of assumptions which work to argue against imbursement: first, that 'mothering' is not work because skills and training are not necessary; second, that people should not be paid if their own needs are being met; third, that carers would anyway be preoccupied in mothering and houseworking; last, as foster care actually enhances family life it does not merit payment. In summary, the more fostering resembles family life the less it should be rewarded. Leat's (1990) study compares payment issues within four groups of financially remunerated carers; child-minders, private agency carers, adult family placement and foster carers. The first three groups felt poorly recompensed but believed that the fact of payment was more important than the amount. Foster carers were in receipt only of allowances and felt that fostering was not so much a 'job' as a way of life. Butler and Charles (1999) discovered that foster carers want improved financial rewards whilst believing that payment for parenting is fundamentally contrary to societal norms.

Thus whilst an understanding of caring is allied to that of family and of altruism there arises an ideology that unpaid caring is qualitatively different and better than paid caring. There is a well-established sociological literature debating this. Formal 'professional' care suggests a wage. Foster carers who register for fee-paying work are selling their private worlds. They are dissolving further the boundaries between the public and the private, between formal and informal care, Ungerson's (1995) 'commodification' of care. Ungerson reviews former debates on whether only informal/unpaid care contains both labour and love and is therefore qualitatively superior. She argues that the belief that care for 'love' is better than for money has implications for women; it could continue to confine them to a sphere that is private, domestic and devalued and thereby sustain the public/private dichotomy. Most carers are female and the payment of low wages rests on the belief that women earn only 'pin money' (Tronto, 1993). But, conversely, some payment may ensure a reasonable supply of carers and thus reinforce this exploitation. Ungerson's argument is that these schemes do not dissolve the boundaries between private and public but strengthen and maintain them. Though in a later paper she proposes that the introduction of payment may attract male employees and lead to a degendering and thereby an upgrading of the status of care (Knijn and Ungerson, 1997).

Most of the literature debating the theory of care discusses care within the family or care of the elderly. Fostering, an exemplar for unpaid care, merits barely a mention whilst continuing to embrace values of philanthropy and unpaid labour. Even in 2004, 56 per cent of local authorities paid their carers below the recommended minimum fostering allowance. Most foster carers have to subsidise the children and experience the dilemma of altruism versus affordability (Oldfield, 1997).

Even though most foster carers are not paid, there are nonetheless expectations of their availability and assumptions about priority to be given, particularly by the female carer, to the needs of the foster child. Carers who have their own children must juggle conflicting demands. Daily life can be dominated by the needs and the timetable of the foster child. Not only must the foster child be cared for but there are statutory reviews and medical checks, and frequently medical treatments. There can be an onerous programme of contact visits with the birth family and the carer's presence may be demanded at meetings or at court. Yet foster carers are not paid to take on all these diverse tasks.

Given both a market economy and a permanent shortage of foster carers, however, there are now various schemes which, in addition to the allowance(s), offer a fee, although never at parity with residential workers. Whereas carers in the formal residential sector are waged with all the obligations but also the contractual rights that this entails, foster carers have no rights but all the obligations. Any 'fee' (which often equates to less than £1 an hour, on the assumption of a single adult with no extra fee for the second carer) purchases round-the-clock care and availability. Although this is a token it introduces an element of payment so that the practical and emotional tasks that foster carers provide for their birth families for free they provide to other children for a fee. Does payment interfere with caring? Does it undermine the ideologies of mothering? Feeling 'rules' are very different in private life and in public life. These foster carers have moved into an area where feeling rules are ambiguous (Nelson, 1990b; Hochschild, 1979).

It is arguable that any payment to foster carers is as a symbol of being valued; it is some sort of recognition that care is 'work'. But waged foster carers are not fully recompensed; their 'symbolic payment' is a consequence of the task and not offered as a rate for the job (Ungerson, 1995). Payment ensures carers' accountability by reinforcing pressures of duty, obligation, altruism and 'love' at an ideological level. The relationship between the care-giver/foster carer and the care-receiver/foster child is thus affected and is commodified (Kirton, 2001a and 2001b). The carer is in receipt of 'a quasi-wages payment for care' (Ungerson, 1995: 39) which is not related to the market rate but is conditional on specific tasks and some sort of contract.

But what else might this fee symbolise? Daily life for foster carers is circumscribed by the demands of bureaucratic caring. Are foster carers compromised as the state purchases the right to interfere and keep them dependent within their own homes? Is the symbolic payment compensation for the fact that birth parents can undermine the authority of foster carers? Have foster carers surrendered to becoming low wage earners rather than altruistic, independent volunteers? Payment certainly purchases public sector access and surveillance. Is it a public statement of the social services department's authority? Carers are neither wholly voluntary nor paid the rate for the job.

Those foster carers in receipt of a fee are treated as self-employed without rights or protection (Shaw and Hipgrave, 1989b). As paid carers, do they regard their status as different from unpaid carers and perhaps consider themselves 'professional' carers? Studies of day-care providers reveal that some of them carved out careers for themselves by implicitly devaluing parental instinct in favour of 'expert' knowledge (Wrigley, 1990; Nelson, 1990a). Although the foundation of their skills was from the same base as the children's mothers and other day-care providers (women's caring), they also claimed an educational expertise for the under fives. Similar differences are found in a comparative study looking at service delivery between mainstream foster carers and specialist foster carer schemes in North America (Unrau, 1994). Whilst unpaid foster carers offered the children their family and warmth and understanding, the paid foster carers perceived their tasks in terms of social training and education. Payment may breed specialism and difference. Rhodes (1993) prophesied that paid schemes could prove divisive and that 'volunteer' foster carers would be viewed as less expert and offering a less specialised care compared to 'paid' colleagues.

Leat and Gay (1987) argue that paid foster caring, because it is underpaid, is exploitative. Market wages for foster carers may prove to be irresolvable. There are sound arguments for paying (foster) carers a fair wage but is this actually affordable? Unpaid carers already give of themselves so much that it 'costs'. There is the physical and emotional stress sometimes intensified by a restricted family and social life (Parker, 1990). There is the cost of forfeiture of employment: estimates in 1982 reckoned loss of earnings to be some £8,500 for each year without taking into account the likelihood of increased expenditure (Mayall and Foster, 1989). External adverse factors impact upon caring since the quality depends upon working conditions, carers' self-esteem and recognition of their work by others (Ungerson, 1990); all of this is applicable to foster family households.

Concepts of household, home and family overlap, as demonstrated by a Curtis Inquiry finding: 'There was . . . much greater happiness for the child by boarding out into a family of normal size in a normal home' (Curtis Report, 1946, para. 370). This ably illustrates how concepts and ideologies regarding the ('normal') family are so often taken for granted. In fact, historically and culturally, the family takes many diverse forms and is noted for its social pluralism. Nonetheless, because of its unquestioned assumptions as offering an optimal environment (male breadwinner, female carer and dependent children), family life in contemporary Western society is seen as the best place to rear children. Yet there is evidence that it was not always like that and possibly never was (Voight, 1986).

Nonetheless, Bebbington and Miles' (1990) comprehensive survey comparing the general characteristics of foster carers to a sample of average families from the General Household Survey (GHS) shows that this description of a typical foster family applied to 75 per cent of almost 3,000 foster families, but to only 31 per cent of the 8,500 families in the GHS. Thus the majority of foster carers appeared to represent the ideology of the nuclear family. The survey reveals a discrepancy of bureaucratic, substitute care not replicating families in the community, but fortifying images of traditional families. Sinclair and colleagues' surveys (2004) show that the majority of foster care households are still couple families with one adult at work and the other at home. Local authorities, through their choice of families, may be reinforcing a conventional family life form although the children in the looked after system will rarely have come from this. Nelson (1994) found that her day-care providers were all aware of the disparity of backgrounds that their charges came from, yet all described a common, established notion of 'family' experience that denied these differences. The social care departments represent the establishment, and the general culture prescribed by central government could be described as middle class. The children within the looked after system come from some of the most poor and disadvantaged families with very limited options. Many foster families may be offering children an experience which is completely incongruent with their birth lives, both because of their own foster family culture but more because of the wishes and demands of the social services.

Smart attests that there is a culture to continue previous efforts to transform disadvantaged/working-class families, lone-parent families and families of people of colour into middle-class idealised families. She argues that the aim is to recapture the time when 'the family' was the solution to all problems; that 'idealised and frozen moment which approximates to the 1950s', in order that families should again represent values of altruism and unpaid labour (1997b: 302). If the majority of foster families map onto this 'idealised and frozen moment', are they portraying an 'unreal' life? Real life demonstrates that families are infinitely variable. In a bid to unpack the concepts surrounding family Morgan (1985) discusses these as having three aspects, which he lists as: the imagery and the complex ideologies, for example the notion of the 'idealised haven'; the actual physical setting, 'the temple of the hearth'; and kinship relationships including the significance of children.

Ideologies of family involve notions of privacy, femininity and of reproduction. There is an expectation that 'real' carers should always be available within the home, though Cheal (1991) reviews the literature that debates family as an antisocial institution which imprisons women. Rich (1977) argues that current social arrangements around the institution of motherhood means that it becomes a central identity for the majority of Western women. Are female foster carers trapped by these structures, or do they regard mothering as empowering[4] and use fostering as a vehicle to emancipation?

The issue is not that women care for children but how this family responsibility gets allocated. Borchorst (1990) argues that biologically motherhood terminates with weaning; any extension is politically constructed, supported by the conceptual public/private divisions. Yet foster carers can 'mother' a series of children for 20 or 30 years. Harris (1977) contends that the strains of (public) life so deny people expression of their talents that they compensate by overloading the (private) family with expectation. Whereas work is about rationality and alienation the family is seen to be about solidarity, companionship and enrichment. The family becomes the only source of fulfilment for most adults who live through their children and therefore make greater emotional demands upon them. Oakley (1979) writes of the importance of children to a mother's feelings of self-esteem (achievement, being wanted and owning property). In Boulton's study (1983), two-thirds of her women found a sense of meaningfulness through their roles as mothers. Some of this may map onto life-as-foster-carer.

Caulfield (1977) suggests that family life for the housewife is more complex. The family is indeed a source of fulfilment but when members are physically not in the home the wife/mother can feel empty, degraded and isolated. Do foster carers want children in order to keep the home full and busy? Are their lives solely, mainly, or occasionally constructed around other people's children? Many of Nelson's day-care providers selected that occupation because it allowed them to remain at home all day with their own children (1990a). They specifically chose to define themselves as mothers who were committed to mothering as a primary role.

Ideologically, households are private and thus able to protect vulnerable children from the dangers of the outside world, though gradually child rearing has become increasingly controlled by the public sphere (Hendrick, 1990). The rationale for this is that the child is a product which must meet exact specifications and that mothers are ignorant (Jagger, 1983). Thus the mother's expertise in the, supposed, privacy of her own house is regularly questioned (Beck-Gernsheim, 1992) and her abilities increasingly the concern of public authorities (Ribbens, 1992). Pascall (1997) emphasises that although family has lost its control it has not lost its functions. It remains the main locus for the care of dependants but many traditional female tasks are now defined and managed from outside the household, by male civil servant managers. Yet, ideologically, home remains 'the principle source of personal fulfilment and identity' (Kumar, 1997: 206) and has considerable significance. To be without a family is to be seen as greatly deprived. Foster care may be about (ful)filling this deprivation of family experience.

Family, together with concepts concerning household, public and private, and care, plus their distinctive gender components, overlap at most points. It has been difficult to discuss any of them as discrete concepts. All have mapped onto our knowledge of foster care only to reveal its paradoxes. Foster families seem to epitomise the ambiguities of family life, the complexities of public and private domains and the multiple conflicting components around the concepts of paid and unpaid care. Foster carers have to manage all these boundaries. Any theoretical overview might suggest that foster care cannot work! Yet we know that it is a favoured institution. Foster carers provide a public service within a private setting, but managed from outside. Although they are called 'carers', children are placed with them in order to have a positive experience of parenting and family life. But relationships within the family are ambiguous. Priority has to be given to the foster children's birth families and foster children have rights that are not necessarily so explicit for carers' own children. Life for foster carers demands many social work skills (Freiburg, 1994) yet the majority remain unpaid whilst also financially subsidising public children. Meanwhile, there is some evidence that local authorities, ignoring the protean nature of family life forms, continue to select 'traditional' families for the care of other people's children.

Family discourse, the language of family life, helps us to understand the family in relation to ourselves and to others. Everyday reality is produced through how people think and talk about activities and relationships. Family is therefore both a concrete set of social ties and sentiments and a socially constructed phenomenon which derives meaning from its context (Gubrium and Holstein, 1990). We all experience family as 'real', but how different are different people's realities? How 'different' are the families of foster carers and how do they experience family life looking after other people's children? If a sense of family is constructed then this leads to an assumption that family is not just biological but can be social/psychological as well. The important understandings of family care could potentially be created between adults and children who are not related. This book is an explanation of foster carers' lives; it is a qualitative study of their portrayal of their varied social practices in order to understand how they 'do' foster care. It is about their perceptions and their world view; it is an account of family-according-to-foster-carers.

3 Dealing with dilemmas: private and personal

Foster 'parents' are now foster 'carers'; a change which confirms and encourages a (re)positioning of foster carers' attitudes vis-à-vis the children. Yet many foster families look after the children for significant periods during the important years of childhood and thereby fulfil a parental role. Additionally legal and current political discourse has shifted to emphasise that parenthood is 'for life'; this has therefore increased the ambiguities for foster carers as quasi-parents.

This chapter discusses how carers manage these ambiguities and the tensions of living as themselves, with their own blood families, whilst simultaneously looking after other people's children. It looks at how the study carers manage those parts of their social worlds which might be described as both 'private' and 'personal'. Although neither are straightforward concepts, they are useful in this context. They aid description of those parts of foster families' lives which are separate from their interactions with the 'external/public' world of the local councils and the foster children's birth families, and help to analyse how they manage the predicament of carer versus parent. This will be examined through the issues they raise regarding time and place and what they say about their subjective experience of their natural/birth parent status compared to their professional/foster carer status. Foster carers have to draw these boundaries in different ways at different times whilst coping with many complex shifts. This chapter considers their accounts of how these (emotional) tensions are managed.

Each study carer was invited to talk about themselves and their lives before they became involved with fostering. This was to give them an opportunity to ground themselves in a life apart from foster care and to put caring into their own context. In fact eight carers chose to start their autobiographies from when they began to foster. They presented their accounts as though the years before were, by comparison, inconsequential; as though their foster carer experiences comprised their significant lives. Becoming a foster carer was for them an epiphanal moment. Although the majority introduced themselves via their childhood experiences, several articulated an explicit awareness that the effect of foster care coloured everything: 'It changes, you know, your life, and I think that social services, social workers forget that you have got a life apart from them and the child that you are looking after' (Louise). When asked if fostering had changed her life, Emma's reply echoed this theme: '*Complete!*[1] Completely turned it topsy turvy and it was our first placement and, and at the end of a few days Gordon and I both said "we can't do this!"'. Louise and Emma are demonstrating some resistance to the way that the local authority's expectation of life-as-foster-carer is to have no other life outside this activity. The change from life-as-it-was to life-as-foster-carer can be so radical that they describe some desire to return to their past, established equilibrium. For them, all life has become life-as-foster-carer.

Ruth unpacks some of the change for her and much of this resonates with the accounts given by others:

> I think the level of involvement they wanted from me in *all* areas was a surprise. Because I just assumed that I was going to just care for this child. To do it quietly in my home. Plod along in my own sweet way but then, have to take these children to contacts[2] and fetch these children from contact and have natural parents in my home ... it was ... a shock. The invasion, I felt at the beginning that it was an invasion of my home, of my lifestyle I suppose, to have to alter this to suit other people which I've *never ever* done before in my life. I'd always lived my life *my* way. Yes, yes and had to change it to accommodate these people.

These quotations demonstrate how foster family life is experienced as markedly different from previous (family) lives. There are many taken-for-granted assumptions about family life, importantly that it is a bounded unit; it has external boundaries. But Ruth's experience is that these have been breached; she has been 'invaded'. She is having to accommodate the expectations and demands of the local council's wishes regarding the foster children within her own household. Like Louise, Ruth states elsewhere in the interview, 'I mean it's not just fostering, it's ordinary extended family commitments as well, you know'. Life-as-foster-carer must exist with life-as-it-was/is. Fostering is one part of their lives alongside other activities but being a foster carer brings change, and change may impact upon life outside foster care.

Some of the changes described by the carers are physical ones to their living conditions. Mandy explains about making the house childproof with plug guards and:

> [W]e didn't have any banisters ... But she [Family Placement social worker[3]][4] said when she came to look, to sort of safety check, she said, 'oh you'll have to get banisters back on the stairs' and it cost us two hundred pounds ... and it was assumed you know, once you were sort of registered. We didn't have the spare two hundred pounds

hanging round for the banisters . . . The decorating, the room costs, and we had to move people around to get the room, you know, so that costs money as well.

For Mandy and her husband, becoming foster carers involved change at a financial cost. It was only after their registration as new carers that the local council demanded new banisters and a decorated bedroom. Although it was difficult for them to raise the necessary monies they nonetheless did so in order to care for a foster child. Like other foster carers they accept the necessity of change and comply. Frances and Alfred independently state that they are prepared to physically modify their house if 'it is the wrong sort of home' (Alfred), whilst Ruth, criticised by the local authority for her standards of cleanliness, first purchases a dishwasher and then:

We took walls out and doors out, lifted carpet because it's *so* unhygienic. For about four years I was in perpetual potty training . . . So I decided that carpets were *most* unhygienic and so just took them and polished the floors which actually makes life much simpler.

Like several other carers she permanently changes her house for the benefit of the foster children. For these carers the effects of fostering upon their way of life is actually visible. Foster care has physical and tangible effects. Whilst Hanneke is having the house extended to better accommodate foster children, Janet is trying to exchange her two-bedroom flat for a three-bedroom house in the village. Mo, who has a company house for his family, persuades his employers to pay for an extension so that they can accommodate Lindsey (seriously disabled) full time rather than for just respite care.[5] For these people life-as-foster-carer requires their active agency in cement(ing) change to their homes.

Gordon tells the sisters that they are fostering, 'it's your house' as though in some sort of gesture of inclusion. Celia, explaining how she encouraged one lad not to vandalise property, says to him, 'that the house he was living in although it wasn't his house but it was his *home* . . . and he should treat it as his home'. So although the foster carers may own the bricks and mortar they are inviting the foster children to share and to participate in their perception and their construction of a notion of 'home'. But the doing of this may result in an 'invasion', as articulated by Ruth, and also specific changes to customs and routines.

Several mention how fostering impacts on their time. Tricia refers to thrice weekly contact in her home as 'really tying'. Janet feels that her care of/being with her foster child should take precedence over attendance at her slimming club and meals with her husband. She also gives priority to social care meetings on market days; all had been part of her usual schedule. Meg adapts her routine to suit the needs of teenage lads who sleep during the day but want to talk into the small hours at night whilst Lenin goes to bed earlier in order to ensure that he is up in time for his foster lad's court appearances. Life/time may now be dictated by the needs of the foster child.

Changes in routines may also result in loss of control as carers discover the dilemma of bureaucratic time versus current, child-centred time. Foster carers offer 24-hour, unscheduled, child-focused care whereas social workers operate on bureaucratic nine-to-five days. Celia expands on the difficulties of maintaining past practice: 'You've got to be able to drop everything and go. Like for instance, we don't plan ahead very often because, sometimes things don't work out'. Sinclair and colleagues (2004) note that fostering impacts upon leisure. For the study carers, timetables and activities are dictated by bureaucracy, the needs of the social care department and the foster children. As these are not always known or predictable, foster carers have their non-foster-carer-lives on hold, in readiness for adaptation to their lives-as-foster-carers. But whilst blood children offer infinity, fostered children can only offer the here and now and uncertainty; they may be here today but tomorrow is unknown, as discussed by Hope below. Foster carers, like Celia, live in the present. The demands of the present, however, can also affect male carers as evidenced in their accounts; fostering impacts upon work lives.

Mike has twice had to leave work in order to look after the foster child whilst his wife, Louise, attends meetings. He has taken days off to attend court and give evidence about the child. Simon alters shifts and, if necessary, forgoes overtime opportunities to attend social care meetings. Brian has changed his job so that he can finish at 2 pm and support Tricia. Similarly Harry works the early shift in order to help Celia with the foster children but even then there are times when this is not sufficient:

> Like taking them to hospital,[6] I got to come home, leave work, take Celia up there, come back again and then go back to work . . . or I'll probably take a day off, instead of losing the money. You know, easier.

Chapter 1 noted that many foster families model a notion of a traditional nuclear family; a male wage earner with a female carer at home. Although some of these foster families may map onto this model, these particular men fulfil more than the wage-earning role. All of them, including Mo cited below, regard their wives as the primary carers and describe themselves as taking secondary, supportive roles. Yet for them it is, as expounded by Harry, like 'having two jobs at one time' and this may therefore have more in common with feminist theories of women who work 'the second shift'.[7] The following extract from Gordon (who is self-employed and whose wife also has paid employment) portrays the dilemmas for him whilst also demonstrating the importance of adaptability:

> [T]he hard part is adjusting my work. I think that's harder because I have to be here some of the time, whereas I'm not saying I'd rather be out

there, I've been *used* to being out there so I've had to change and say 'no I've got to be in here and I've got to change my times. Whereas I could be out at 8 o'clock in the morning I can't be out until 9 o'clock'. That kind of thing which is not a big deal, but it's the biggest thing that I've found.

He further explains that he is postponing plans to develop his business as he has decided that this would be in conflict with his availability to care for the foster children. In fact, when caring for two demanding fostered brothers, he worked only two days out of the ten. In interview he reflects whether he should permanently work part time in order to better look after the foster children. For Gordon work and income have had to adjust to the demands of foster care. Foster care has become such an imperative that the necessity of earning his living takes second place and Emma is now the main wage earner. Emma is supportive of this; like Gordon she wishes to ensure that their lives-as-foster-carers retain priority.

Much of this resonates with Mo and Hope's situation. She too has paid work. Of his own career Mo explains:

I had opportunity to do more within the Company, go up the ladder . . . now I cannot commit myself to more than what I do . . . The new post would take me further up the ladder and accept more responsibility . . . It does mean I'm more hours of work . . . I wouldn't like that you know. I like to be here at 3 o'clock if Hope can't make it, because Lindsey's taxi [from school] will be here. You know I cannot really commit myself.

He can commit to the fostered child but not to his career. Elsewhere he relates how he discusses with his manager, accepting demotion in order to ensure that he can be more available for Lindsey should Hope be delayed. Mo presents his life-as-foster-carer role to be more important than his life-as-bread-winner role. These male carers make sacrifices in order to support the care of foster children. In these instances caring and economic imperatives are related and provide new rationales for action. Like Morgan's 'new men' (1996) and Neale and Smart's separated fathers (2000), who continually re-assess their work lives in light of the changing needs of the children together with the circumstances of the other parent, some male foster carers organise their time around fostered children.

There are other experiences regarding balancing the demands of home and work. Georgina, a new carer, finds the mix of life-as-wage-earner and life-as-foster-carer difficult to manage. Her employment does not lend itself to the flexibility and adaptability previously noted as required for fostering. The family had offered weekend respite to a child originally in boarding school, only to find that when circumstances changed, the social care staff expect them to be his full-time carers:

[I]nterfering with my work has been too much . . . [fostering] is interrupting my work day and, my own children I don't think about them . . . I don't have to worry about them from when I walk out the door to when I come in at night, and that's not the case with Dylan because alright he's fostered, 'cos they're ringing you, they're making arrangements, it's his assessment in another month, it's this, that and the other.

Georgina's life as a career woman is important to her. She experiences this as being in conflict with her life as a foster carer and has difficulties with the accommodation. Foster care impinges upon and interferes with her working day. Unlike Mo she does not want to give her life-as-foster-carer precedence but is determined to retain her career. She is used to keeping separate her life-as-mother and life-as-worker; foster care does not fit these demarcations but spills into work and erodes her boundaries. Her pursuit of career/self-development creates conflicts with social care's notions of duty and responsibility for Dylan's needs. Generally most of the carers, and particularly the new carers, find fostering to be more demanding than anticipated but Georgina alone is open about her resistance. She objects to the local authority's demands encroaching on her work-life which she wants ring-fenced from her life-as-foster-carer.

Life-as-foster-carer can also be problematic for carers' social lives. Frances ruminates on some of the changes that she and her husband will make for both fostered teenagers and their visiting parents:

I think we have to be adaptable because if they [visiting parents] needed to smoke because they were very nervous or whatever, as a general rule we would prefer people to smoke outside, but I, I personally wouldn't make a fuss about it. But the thing about drink is, is another thing that we've discussed as a family because we've had to talk about this with drugs rehabilitation and if you've got somebody with you who's alcoholic I think it's important to get rid of all the alcohol in your home and we would be willing to do that . . . it wouldn't be an enormous problem, I'd rather do that than run the risk of somebody being tempted.

She and Alfred are prepared to change their social habits in order to foster. Like others in this study they construct themselves as having to adapt and change in order to accommodate other people's children. If necessary, as in this example, change will be explicit in behaviour.

Changing behaviours may impinge on social networks. Both Tricia and Harry mention the difficulties of answering friends' and neighbours' questions about foster children when the information is confidential to the child. Harry uses the word 'embarrassing' since friendship is frequently based on openness whereas foster carers are instructed not to explain. Several of the narratives demonstrate that being a foster carer can affect social life as carers have to erect new boundaries whilst dismantling old ones. Hanneke's experience is that badly behaved children are not welcome in the homes of friends whilst Stan finds that a houseful of foster children is just too many for invitations to Sunday lunch. Harold (a new carer with his first foster child, Ruby) explains how he makes choices about visiting relatives with her:

> My mother's birthday yesterday, I sent her some flowers . . . but I will have to go over by myself. I don't want to take Ruby over there because she'll [his mother] ask her embarrassing questions. 'Why are you staying with Kathleen? [his wife]' . . . And I don't want her to put Ruby in that position.

So whereas, in the past, he and Kathleen had taken his elderly mother out for a birthday lunch, this year he sends flowers and will take a day off work in order to visit on his own. His life-as-foster-carer has modified his behaviour in his life-as-son. Emma's still new experience as a foster carer causes her to surmise that 'you would have to probably match what (foster) placement you had to what, to what friends you visited'. Kelly expounds on the complexities of social events with their foster boys. Family and friends are:

> [N]ot as sensitive as we are. Clive [husband] and I are very, very sensitive to our boys' feelings . . . and we try and help them to join in, and make conversation with them. But I don't think other people think like that . . . some of them are really, really nice. I suppose some aren't quite as under-standing. Like some people say, 'Why do you put up with it? [abusive behaviour] You're absolutely mad' . . . You either do put up with it or you make them [foster children] move out which you try and avoid. You don't want that at any cost. You try and stick with them, and help them but we've had a lot of comments like 'You're absolutely mad' or 'I wouldn't have my home, no one would damage my home like that' . . . I find it very hurtful and it's easier to get on with people now who do foster. I prefer to go out with people who foster . . . They've been in that position, they're understanding, they know what it's like.

In line with the narratives of several other carers, Kelly's account of look-ing after other people's children is that, as far as her social life is concerned, her life-as-foster-carer must come first. This involves more redrawing of boundaries. Those friends and members of the family who are not able to empathise with life-as-foster-carer are considered uncaring, not only to the fostered children but also towards herself. Her personal identity is bound up in her foster carer status. She and Clive interpret this as a commitment to continue to care for fostered children even when, as in their case, children have verbally threatened or physically attacked both them and their house. Her belief in the priority of her life-as-foster-carer means that she has become gradually disillusioned with past friends in favour of other foster carers who share her convictions and her experiences. Olivia, reflecting on past friends, concludes, 'you tend to lose that normality'. Life-as-foster-carer can be so 'topsy turvy' that foster carers estrange themselves from old friends/the past life-as-it-was and reassure themselves with others in the foster care world of the present who understand 'why you are dealing with children that are kicking you and punching you and swearing at you' (Olivia). New boundaries of empathy and understanding only come from those who share the identity; fostering becomes a new and central care identity.

The decision to foster affects not just the adults but their children and the extended family. Kelly, Keith, and Lionel are examples of the many carers who talk of grandmothers and adult children being 'police checked' so that they can babysit the foster children. None of them intimate that this is in any way strange or different from how all families manage a social life. For all of them it has become a taken-for-granted fact. Most of the foster carers talk of their relatives as simply accepting and absorbing the foster children into the extended family; the most usual evidence being the parity of gifts between all children of the household. Hanneke states, as though it should be expected, that both her ex-husband and his mother always send Christmas presents for all the children, birth and fostered. Even where there has been initial reluctance from elderly relatives, carers state that this had been overcome and greetings cards are now sent to foster children signed 'Nan' and 'Grandpa'. There is little anticipation from the carers that extended family members might have contrary views about relationships being hijacked for children who are not related, only an expectation that they should accept elective family relationships which then redefine family obligations. Neither is there, in general, any regard to the views of fostered children's birth relatives who may not wish to be replaced.

Nevertheless, there are signs of extended (foster) family resistance. Mandy's mother was 'very concerned . . . worry for me and my health', but when she telephoned 'Timmy [foster child] answered and actually she was very supportive and she's rung me since . . . Now it has happened I think she'll be alright' (Mandy). Mike's mother's reaction was similar, 'I don't think she was very happy at all . . . I think it was concern for us really. "You've got three children of your own, why do you want to bring another one up?" but she's fine with Victoria [foster child]'. Here any lack of enthusiasm is presented as concern for the foster carers themselves rather than any reluctance of kin to become involved in fictive blood relation-ships with children who are not blood relatives. Generally the majority of accounts indicate that the speaker's own zeal for, and commitment to, foster care is so total that there is no space for the doubts of others. Both these extracts suggest that the foster children were instrumental in the conver-sion and as Cyril points out: '*Your* friends they're gonna meet him [foster child] and you want 'em to like him as well him to like them'. This suggests that, for Cyril, his foster child is so much part of the family that it matters to him that Craig is not just acceptable but also actively likeable in the eyes of those who matter, his friends. Although a minority of the carers consider the children's birth families relevant, the general focus is on incorporating the foster child into the foster family. In this respect foster carers can be powerful.

Although 'family' is a much-contested site there are several notions that hold firm in Western ideology. It is regarded as a social unit comprising adults and children with all children given the same status. There are differentials within the category of child in terms of age and gender but studies of step families (Ribbens McCarthy and Edwards, 2002) demonstrate that 'fairness' is a key theme and a barrier to further demarcation. Comparative analysis reveals strong parallels in the subjective experiences of step families and of foster families.

Almost all the carers are adamant in their response to the vignette concerning the boss's invitation excluding the two foster children[8] that they must always be included and receive complete parity with carers' own birth children. Ruth admits that she had attended a family wedding without a foster child but had ensured that all were aware of her disagreement and anger. Typically the statements of the carers are that all children living in the household should be treated the same, whatever their status. Although they may have dual roles as foster carers and as birth parents, most of them want to be perceived as able to present the same persona and offer similitude to all children in the foster family. The following extract from Brian's interview encapsulates some of the ambiguities of this situation:

> [Y]ou're not supposed to be a parent are you? You're not supposed to be replacing a parent. You're supposed to be a carer looking after them, not a *parent* . . . I called myself a foster parent and I still do *now* but I suppose . . . you're *being* the parent to them but you're *not* their parent! I mean I don't really know, because you're not trying to eliminate their parent from them and you're not trying to replace their parent, *but* you're trying to give them what most other children have got and that *is* a parent who they live with and is looking after them.

Brian struggles to make sense of the (internally experienced) similarities and differences of parenting and foster caring but argues that he gives all children the same; a position taken by some stepfathers in reconstituted families. Brian is being the parent to them all but as Grace's extract also demonstrates, parental parity is not possible:

> Grow them as you grow your own children because there's no difference between it really. It's just that you're not the mum but everything else is just the same to *me* . . . to me they was my children. They weren't any difference . . . except if my children do anything wrong I give them a

clout round the ears. You know, a touch round the ear which I wouldn't do, not that it would be wrong but somebody might say 'well because they're not your children you're hitting them'. And I would not like anybody to think that because I wouldn't school a child because it's not mine. I would school them exactly how I school my children . . . It's just children need looking after . . . feed them, bath them . . . and *love*, love, the most important thing is to be able to love somebody else's child as you would love your own . . . And they're *all* my children, no matter whose child they are.

This last sentence neatly summarizes the contradictions and the complexities of the foster carer's (parental) identity. Although Grace thinks that she is the same person to both her own children and to any foster children, upon reflection she realises that she cannot treat both groups with parity. Although the feeling and the meaning may be the same, the techniques must be different. Foster carers are expressly forbidden to physically chastise any foster child so Grace cannot, as she would with her own, 'give them a clout round the ears'. Again, this reflects themes in studies on stepfamilies regarding discipline; it can be exercised with 'your own' because of underlying assumptions of love and obligation (Ribbens McCarthy *et al.*, 2000). This is problematic for Grace since an explicit and integral part of her caring is 'schooling'/disciplining children and it is important that she is seen by others to administer the same standards of care/'schooling' to all children. Sanctions for foster children are very proscribed and she describes, elsewhere, how she therefore talks to them about their behaviour. Nonetheless the differences are a source of concern for her so she falls back upon the fact that she loves all the children in the household with parity.

These ambiguities about fairness abound within the foster carers' accounts. Examination reveals the complexities; that it is not actually possible to guarantee total equality of care within the household given the differences in status between the children. The adults do have to act as parents to birth children and as foster carers to the children of others. There is, for example, some concern for the foster child's physical well being. Mike's extract illustrates some of this:

[W]e've got a patio and I don't like Victoria [foster child] playing on the slide . . . you don't want her to injure herself. I'm not saying I want my children to be injured but there's a difference of taking a foster child to the hospital to have a stitch put in their head . . . whereas I'd p'raps allow my children to do it, if they had a bump they had a bump, or a graze. But you really don't want Victoria to go to meet her mum with a big graze on her leg . . . I think that's another sub-conscious thing that you do, it's not an intentional thing . . . but you definitely do . . . Part of growing up is to get the odd bump and graze but you really don't want it to happen to, it wouldn't do them any harm, but it's what other people portray as, 'Well why wasn't you watching her?' Well probably the same reason as I wasn't watching my own daughter.

Mike has ownership of and authority over his own daughters but not for Victoria. This anxiety regarding bureaucratic surveillance and the external 'g(r)aze' resonates with Mandy's statement:

[Y]ou've got to protect yourself from the same allegations [as those from the social care agency against the birth family] and so now I'm so protective of Timmy, even if he falls over or he's got a bruise you know they're gonna think it's me . . . Even though I've been nursing a long time and I know all about accountability and I've had some cases of abuse and things and I've been one of the professionals dealing with it . . . on the other side. I just feel a bit vulnerable not being a professional doing this.

Mandy feels the difference; risk at work is protected by professional status. Within the home she is a maternal/informal carer. Risk at home leaves her exposed. Both these carers are new and have attended training courses on allegations of abuse and neglect against foster carers. Like all carers they are aware of their vulnerability should the child they look after come to any harm. Care is most obvious when it is lacking. Whereas Mike encourages his three young daughters to further feats of physical prowess, he is mindful of actually inhibiting any foster child. Mandy, as a qualified nurse, feels competent about dealing with cases of abuse in her 'professional' capacity but as a foster carer in her own home she states that she is deskilled. In these circumstances foster carers treat their birth children and the children of others not with parity but with difference.

Nonetheless there are instances of the ways in which carers instil parity. Keith reports that it feels odd when the 4-year-old foster child calls him Keith and his 22-year-old son calls him 'Dad'. In most cases the social care department actively discourage the use of parental nomenclature so it becomes problematic when Timmy decides to copy their son and call Keith and Mandy 'Dad and Mum'. Keith and Mandy's response is to ask their son Robin to use their first names so that Timmy will not feel the difference. Here it would seem that, in order to impose parity, their roles as foster carers take precedence over those of parents to their own child/blood.

Whatever the protean form of family, fairness with regards to children is considered a major issue. Most carers in this study wish to offer parity to all children within the household. If Yvonne buys a gift for a grandchild she also purchases for the foster children. Jackie insists that her three fostered young people have to abide by exactly the same conditions as her son. Mo wants for his foster child the same responsibility, with its potential for authority, that he has for his birth children. In general most carers say that foster children are equal to their own blood children and insist that the terms and conditions for living within the household are non-discriminatory. They love them 'like their own' explaining that the foster children, although not the same as their own, merit equality of treatment. Fairness within family is sacrosanct.

Yet, set against this, foster carers struggle with the notion that the foster child's needs, on occasions, have to be regarded as paramount. There may be conflict between competing family interests as foster children's needs take precedence over birth children. This is epitomised by Mike's response (in line with the majority of carers) to the vignette posing the carer's dilemma of attendance at birth children's school concert or foster child's court case: 'my gut feeling is saying that I have to go with my son and watch the concert, but as a foster carer you're saying "no"'. As Ali Shah says, 'we know our duty'. Duty to the fostered child means that they will forgo their children's concert. Most carers responded with, 'there would be other concerts'. Some recalled personal experience of similar situations, with the majority giving the foster child priority.

Many re-frame this moral dilemma with the explanation that as the foster children came from such sad beginnings they deserve better, if not the best. They wish to ensure for the foster children the 'proper childhood' they believe their own children have experienced. Mary identifies that, 'it's natural, you get a kid who's been hurt, you want to do everything to, you know, take the pain away, show them that there are nice people in this world . . . we all do it . . . "My [birth] child's alright he's, he's had all this"'. Brian teases out the dilemma;

> I try hard and I don't think I treat them any differently . . . My children . . . have said more than once, '*They* get away with far more than we were ever allowed to'. So you have to sort of be a bit *tactful* and say, 'Well, you had a decent home and you were brought up, you know, bit better so the fact that these children . . . may not have had the same advantages that *you've* had. And you've got to take that into allowance. I mean that's all there is to it. Not everybody's been as lucky as you, to have had a mum and dad to look after you all the time. Sometimes you've got to remember that'. And, on the whole . . . they [his birth children] have put up with a lot.

Brian says that he treats the foster children with parity but actually constructs them as different, more needy than his own three and mediates this inequality to them. There are rules for his children but different, individual rules for fostered children.

For couples without birth children there can be different family dilemmas. John and Ann, describing a 'quasi-adoption' foster situation offering permanency to two brothers actively reflect on the nature of their care. They experience 'all the feelings that you have when you've brought up your own

children and . . . would be totally distraught if the placement broke down'
but decide that:

> [S]ince they *were* seeing their *real* mother and father and their sister . . .
> and we didn't actually *feel* like their parents and we have made a con-
> scious decision that we would try to respect *their* lifestyle . . . So we
> have very much viewed it that we are *not* the parents because we feel if
> we try to be their parents they will actually lose something of great
> value . . . I feel like neither a parent nor a carer. I probably feel more
> like a *step*-parent than I do either of those things.

Ann's interview demonstrates some ambivalence about parent/carer status.
She has experienced all the feelings that parents have and would be
'distraught' to lose the boys. However, they have an active connection with
their birth family and this preserves the 'gap' for her and she therefore cate-
gorises herself as neither parent nor foster carer but opts for a parent at one
hand removed, a step-parent. She has organised the tension and made it
manageable. There is no guarantee that children placed long term with
foster carers will remain. Control over movement remains primarily with
the local councils and, occasionally, with the children themselves though
sometimes foster carers request removal. Ann, aware of this, explains elsewhere how important her career and outside work is in order to spread the
emotional risk and prevent her from becoming 'submerged' in fostering.
It is as though there is a danger of her identity being drowned by foster
care and she maintains her work as a lifejacket, a device in order to retain
her other essential self.

   All the study carers find different ways of coping with the tensions around
the expressive aspects of including foster children within their families. The
majority of children in foster care are placed short term so mostly the
carers talk about the problems of emotional involvement and the subsequent
pain at parting. Celia uses contact, in this case the regular but frequently
inconvenient visits of the foster baby's grandparents, as a helpful distancing
mechanism:

> I think it's very important that Micah gets to know them so therefore
> I don't mind and also I don't want to get too attached to him . . . So
> when his grandma and grandpa come I sit back and I let them take
> over . . . So in a way I really don't mind that [the visits].

Kathleen explains how she is attempting not to become overly involved with
Ruby: 'We're trying very hard to keep our distance and not rushing to kiss
her goodbye when she goes to school . . . I'm trying, trying not to be over
affectionate, but if she wants it, it's there'. She confirms the emotional risk
both to herself, her husband and to the foster child. This extract suggests
that it is difficult for the foster carers to hold this emotional boundary; the

affection for Ruby is readily available. She hints that the managing of this boundary is dictated by the foster child; if Ruby wants the emotion/affection then the foster carers will meet this need.

Similarly Mike muses on the fact that they have become too fond of/ involved with their foster child. He anticipates much sadness when she leaves and wants to prevent a recurrence:

> I'm not saying we'll do things differently next time but, as long as you've got it in your mind . . . you have to put it as a *job* I think, rather than getting too personally involved and we are with Victoria . . . especially Louise [wife] . . . Yeah, try to, whether it will be possible or not I don't know, not, not that it will in a way that will affect the child, but to try and be a bit harder if you like, more of a shell.

In contrast to Grace who emphasises the importance of loving the children, Mike considers constructing a boundary, an emotional shell, between himself and future foster children. He anticipates some sort of changes in behaviour and attitudes in order to protect himself and his wife, but ones that will not affect the future foster children. He suggests that they could adopt the mind-set of fostering being a 'job', as though the concept of work involves less sentiment, or at least tighter emotion management.

Janet uses the same analogy in order to manage this same 'detached attachment' with Craig. She posits, 'You're holding back that little bit every time, which is a shame because I still feel he would achieve more, you know [if I didn't]'. She describes the complexities of maintaining this emotional boundary between herself and Craig.

> It would come back to this part again of getting too involved . . . I think it's safer to . . . class it as a job. Although I suppose the job satisfaction part of it is the fact that Craig's happy and at the end of the day I'm, *I'm hoping that I've achieved something with him that he can move on to his next place* . . . and say 'well, Janet gave me so and so and I, I learned a lot'. So that would be to me job satisfaction and I'd feel that I'd done a good job . . . There's always that little bit, you're standing back, but as I say you, you do understand and they do understand, but it does make the job a little bit harder.

Elsewhere she perceives that her emotional attachment to foster children cannot be the same as that with her own grandchild. She presents herself as responsive-foster-carer to Craig and emotional-grand-mother to Terry. Musing on the differences she says:

> My behaviour towards Terry is a lot, a lot more open. I can say to Terry 'come here and I'll put your pyjamas on you', whereas with Craig I say 'here's your pyjamas', you know, 'you go and put them on' . . .

> I suppose it was, 'cos you're wearing two hats then if you know what I mean.

Janet would seem to understand and be able to differentiate between the 'two hats' that she must wear, simultaneously, when caring for both boys. She may feel the same about both boys but her behaviour must differentiate. She can be expressive (grand)mother to Terry but must remain, reluctantly, detached foster carer with Craig.

Daisy's interpretation of this difference (detached versus expressive carer) relies upon her personal understanding of the distinction between foster carer and foster mother:

> Oh I liked to be a foster *mum* eventually. I know that doesn't come straight away, but I would like to be a foster mum . . . at the moment I feel just a foster carer 'cos I have them for a very short time and I know I can't bond with them and even if I did you know, it's a very short time it wouldn't be very good for me, it would be too emotional. So I'm just a foster carer for now. But when you're a foster mum is when you've got them for a long time . . . I look forward to being a foster mum, you know dealing with all yeah, the, all the problems and everything that they bring.

This extract suggests that getting emotionally involved with children who are placed short term carries too much emotional risk for the adult who therefore safeguards her position by considering herself as a 'carer'. For Daisy, behaving as a foster carer consists of a particular set of self-protective attitudes and emotions. Set beside this she looks forward to a future when she can behave as a foster 'mum', to bond and to deal with the children in an entirety which includes 'all the problems'. Being a key support in a child's life, being a mum or, in Daisy's instance a foster mum, therefore involves other, different sets of attitudes, emotions and behaviours and will redefine her as a new person offering a different sort of care.

Many of the carers debate the ambiguities of full, expressive caring/loving the foster children. Hope charts the emotional change that occurred with Lindsey who was placed for respite weekends for three years and then became a long-term placement:

> I can't just switch off and do things mechanically for her and I, I love this child as my own daughter . . . it's been such a gradual thing that before you know when, you're besotted by her, you just love her like a daughter, but I couldn't say to you it happened the second year, third, it was just one of these slow things until now, to this point when she's been here a year [full-time] that you know I can feel the warmth in me the same as I think of Arash and Zeeba [birth children] and the warmth it's that, you

know. I'm sure there *must* be some difference, but I can't, I don't *feel* any difference.

Hope raises expectations that biology matters but intimate caring has inevitably led to an individual bond and to love. Others, like Janet and Mike already cited, feel that to hold back emotionally means that, at least, the child will not do as well as they could. Alice, a new carer, talking of her two-year-old foster child says:

> When he first arrived, I suppose I was very hard to myself and I thought, 'right I'm not going to get attached. He's just staying here. I'm not going to get involved to the depths that I can't let him go, he's only staying. I know he's gonna go back. I'm not gonna get that attached that I'm going to get really devastated'. But I can't. You can't *not* get attached . . . I can see the difference. I can see the difference in the way he plays from the first couple of days he was here when I was thinking 'I'm not going to get close' and the way he behaves now. 'Cos before, he'd do something and he would just look at me across the room and then he'd put it down and then he'd go and do something else. Whereas now, he'll do something and he'll come running up to me with his arms up to show me how clever he is and I think if I tried to keep him at a distance he'd know and that just wouldn't be fair on him.

Whilst acknowledging that he 'has to go back' Alice also says, elsewhere in the interview, 'he's mine now', meaning that he is like her own child and that she feels the same authority about him. She also reports that the social care training included reference to children leaving so, as the extract demonstrates, she commenced the placement with a view that she should avoid emotional involvement. But co-residence brings a daily, immediate quality into play; a physical quality – he comes running to her with his arms up – and this has sabotaged her intentions. She thus constructs their particularistic bond in terms of the child's needs and has become emotionally tied. Foster carer training may teach detachment but foster carer daily lived experience invokes attachment. Meg is adamant that 'they all want love' and sees her task as supplying this:

> I think [of] myself as a foster mum. I've *always* thought myself as a foster mum . . . they say foster carer but I don't like it . . . I think to be a carer is like being a, going and sweeping up somebody else's house and looking after that . . . but I think what *all* these kids want, and I don't care whether they are 13-year-old boys or 14-year-old boys or two-year-old children, they just want lots of love. That's all they're missing in their life is love and care.

Love, including overtones of therapeutic love, is hereby defiantly asserted. Meg conflates the giving of unconditional love with, not just her role in fostering, but specifically as a foster mother. This is quite a complex, if not ambiguous, concept as elsewhere in her interview she criticises the birth mothers for not loving their children sufficiently and also explains that the foster children call her Meg 'because they all have their own mothers'. Nonetheless her presentation of the justification of her role is that she does not emotionally withhold from the foster children and that this is tied in with her notions of real motherhood. 'Love' offered by foster carers is part of a public discourse but in this extract Meg affirms the love of private discourse as she manages and measures social motherhood against biological motherhood, usually constructed as real, loving motherhood. Perhaps for her and for others in this study, because their love includes quality of care, the foster carers consider themselves to be more of a mother than the real biological mothers. The birth mothers of the foster children may have loved their children but, as constructed by foster carers, they failed to care adequately for them.

This importance of love is echoed in Margaret's interview. Talking of the school leavers that they foster, she says, 'Well there should be just plenty of love. You want to give those kind of children, 'cos that's what they are, this little boy'. Margaret then goes on to describe how she provides 'plenty of love':

> I cook his dinner, I listen to what he likes to tell me . . . he comes in and puts his little face round the corner, says 'hello' when he comes in and he'll make me a cup of tea . . . yeah that kind of thing you know, that kind of little thing. You don't get hold of them and love them, nothing like that, he's a *boy* . . . Well it's just little things like, that you're there, you know, he can look round and see somebody in the kitchen or somebody about . . . like when I was a child, you could come and find your mum in the kitchen working with the tea or the dining room or wherever you like to be, your mother was *there*.

Like Meg she elides love with motherhood and interprets its presentation, not by a show of physical affection, but through presence; 'being there' equates with love.

However, there are risks for foster carers if they behave as, and allow themselves to feel like, a mother to a child who is not theirs. Attachment brings possibilities for conflict. Upset and angry for the foster child, Georgina 'had a go' at one mother about failed contact arrangements. There are also opportunities for rivalries, some more explicit than others. Georgina expresses regret that their foster child 'doesn't want a cuddle or a kiss . . . his mother says she loves him and he cuddles her and you thought he would' [want Georgina to cuddle him]. Those who do not maintain the emotional barrier between foster carer status and parent status leave themselves vulnerable. Hope, when talking of Lindsey's parents' monthly contact visits, admits that, 'part of me wants to be really selfish and say I wish that three hours didn't happen . . . I'd like to be allowed to get on and care for Lindsey the best way I can'.

Grace, relating her feelings of deep loss when three foster children left her to live with their grandmother, states how they said they would run away back to her, to which she had replied, 'You know what to do, don't you? . . . You just go into a police station and give the police the address and tell them where you want to go and you come. Your room will always be here'. Like Margaret, still 'being there' demonstrates love for the children, though this may raise issues about the risks of permeating the boundaries between foster carer status and its 'professional' behaviours since foster carers are expected to love and to let go. In contrast, parent status, with its differently charged emotional behaviours can, as with Hope, result in rivalry with the children's birth families. Similarly Kelly relates that birth parents, whatever the history of abuse, are all-important for the children. She had not anticipated how 'loyal' the children would be and how the children 'didn't see them as they really were'. Ann, discussing the 'bonds of emotion' between John and herself with the boys concludes, 'but it *isn't* the same thing they give their parents or their parents show to them'. Attachment to children can be painfully problematic.

These carers demonstrate that caring for foster children involves emotional attachment with a risk of painful intensity of feeling. Something of this is conveyed in the following extract from Tricia's interview in which she is talking of a past placement:

> We'd been fostering a little girl for over six years who we thought would stay permanent, who was *extremely* difficult. And that broke down and that was hard. That's the hardest thing I've *ever* had to do. It broke my heart and really, really got to me. I've never felt so *distraught* . . . just unable to cope with the situation, myself. That's really, really hard. And its taken a long time to almost get over that, to the point you know that we actually moved house . . . We really had to go through a slow process of moving on again and rethinking what we could, or perhaps what we wanted to offer in future to safeguard ourselves. *Hopefully* it won't happen again. I think, you know, when you've been through virtually hell and high water for six years and you just put your *all* into that and still, you know.

In this case Marcia had not only made a false allegation of sexual abuse against Tricia's husband, Brian, but had also come between them to the extent that the viability of their marriage was at stake.[9] Tricia's presentation of her situation, like that of other study carers, is that she had not retained any emotional boundaries with this foster child. She had offered Marcia everything so that the child would feel secure with them; she had given her emotional 'all'. Thus, when the placement finishes prematurely, Tricia is bereft. In order to pick up the pieces of their family life she and Brian physically move to a new house that holds no memories of this foster child. This physical, but symbolic action, allows them to emotionally 'move on' and start afresh. This extract typifies both the pain and the extraordinariness of fostering.

Much of Tricia's pain resonates with Hope's recollection of Lindsey's unplanned removal by her birth mother:

> Monday night we got a phone call at half past seven and Lindsey was gone the next day. We're left here to pick up the pieces and it was really like a bereavement. I've never as yet had a bereavement that I've been mature, old enough to understand the intense feelings, until as I say Lindsey was taken back and it was just horrendous . . . sometimes I want to just erase that 'foster' bit and believe that she's my own daughter, but you know, I suppose at the bottom of my heart I know she's, she's somebody else's daughter and I've just got the privilege and whatever to care for her.

For Hope the incident was like a death. Her emotional tie with Lindsey was so intense that, when she was removed by her own birth mother, Hope could not respond as a foster carer. She resists reminding herself, as Brian does, that the children are 'not mine . . . on loan'. Hope would like to believe that Lindsey is her own child. For her, foster carer and mother have become the same. Even though she has to remember that Lindsey is not her own blood child, any boundaries between behaving-as-a-foster-carer and behaving-as-a-mother are now extinguished. But it was not always thus. She did not always feel this way:

> I remember the first time she came for respite. To change her nappy, it really made me cringe to have to do it, cleaning up another person's child, to be honest with you. Although I'm a qualified nurse and I've been doing it, but it's just actually when you move in and you know sort of, it felt really weird. Really *weird* having to change her and getting the boundaries right for physical contact and things like this because again you know you can. There's things that you do quite spontaneously with your own children. But you know because that child's not your child. I don't know, it does *feel* different, or it *did* feel different then, right at the beginning.

This extract shows that foster carers can/do feel differently about foster children and their own children. Hope was physically repelled by Lindsey in carrying out a task that she had undertaken many times for her own children without a problem. She was initially aware of both physical and emotional boundaries ('when you move in . . . it felt really weird') in the care of this child and was disturbed by their ambiguity. Some of this is reflected, though barely and rarely, by other carers. It is as though foster care insists upon the loving acceptance of a child, even if unlovely. Yet Hanneke makes the point that 'the kids, most of them are so difficult they're not easy or *nice* to have', whilst Grace reflects that 'even God's children can be cruel sometimes'. Alfred, still awaiting a first foster placement, ponders, 'we need to be able to tell exactly how we feel about those kids and sometimes you're going to feel like murdering them'. Two carers, speaking about how they cope with difficult behaviour in public, construct a biological boundary between themselves and the foster child. Olivia 'just kept on thinking he actually isn't my child. So that's okay, he's not my child'. In a similar situation Ruth jokes, 'not from my loins!'.

Edwards and colleagues (1999) note class differences of care in step-families: a middle-class emphasis on biological parenting and a working-class acceptance of social parenting. Working-class step-fathers are more inclusive in their emotional and practical attitudes to the children of their new partners. There may be similarities in foster care.

Most of the study carers consider their attitudes and concern for fostered children to be as solicitous and as loving as for their own birth children. Yet, in order to cope, they must make continuous changes for and around the foster children. Looking after the children of others has a significant impact upon their time, space and work life whilst affecting extended families and social friendships. Foster care shapes carers' individualities; there are ambiguities around birth/natural parent identities and also foster carer/professional parent identities so that offering the foster child equality with blood/own children can be problematic. Importantly there are complexities around emotional boundaries; the dilemmas of attachment or detachment.

This examination of how foster carers manage their somewhat precarious worlds has identified the conundrum that, as there are no models for foster care, the families are left to make daily sense of their position and to renegotiate and to re-present themselves in their 'internal' dealings. Bureaucracy may shape the external context of carers' relationships with the children but the internal reality is that fostering becomes a care identity based on love. Thus the many ambiguities around the position of the foster child leads to major dilemmas for the carers in their subjective experience.

4 How foster carers position themselves

The previous chapter focused on how foster carers interpret and cope with incorporating 'other' children into the family and how this affects their ways of being. The analysis continues with how they understand themselves within the contexts and constraints of their foster-carer-lives. It examines their perception of their status vis-à-vis the social care departments, the children's birth parents and also in regard to the foster children. Further constructions are explored: foster carers as rescuers via notions of family and of home; as change agents and as paid agents; as finding opportunities through foster care for expiating past experience; and foster carers as responsible for all facets of children's lives.

Some argue that all families are under scrutiny and therefore semi-public, even if this is part of an internalised public gaze whereby people (covertly) monitor themselves.[1] But for foster families the scrutiny is overt and they could thereby be described as semi-public institutions, held accountable for their actions because strangers (local council staff) have an influence upon them. Some carers comment that social workers are supportive, supply information and training, and that they positively enjoy official visits.

Nonetheless there are more critical and negative statements about the department and its personnel; numerous complaints that the local authority makes them feel distanced, misunderstood and mistrusted. Foster carers believe that the council's bureaucratic systems result in disorganised resources and poor practical arrangements. Generally carers say they are exploited; that the department is intrusive and ignores their outside-fostering lives. They feel undervalued and ill informed, 'they know lots of things, but it's always been "us and them"'. Stan's complaint is echoed by Lenin who has been asked to undertake a task beyond his competence – supporting a young person at the police station:

> I might be the only one in the whole world that has this gripe . . . I might've *offended* everybody so much that they turn round and say 'right we'll make it a little bit harder for him', but the point surely has to be for anybody . . . we need support. Foster carers need support

now, it's no good throwing me in the deep end saying 'you're now an appropriate adult'.

The perceptions of Stan and Lenin are that the local authority is unhelpful and unsupportive. Lenin wonders if he is in some way responsible for the behaviour of the social workers. The dominant culture of the social care department is seen, by them, as very powerful whilst their position is portrayed as powerless. Several recount similar incidents. Mike's experience of social services training is 'not in touch with the reality of what really happens in foster care and they were saying the support you get is paramount and, and it's not, it's not there'.

Mike recounts how his family was so distressed by the baby's reactions to contact that he telephoned the manager who promised action but, 'nothing changed . . . you get to the point where you say, "come and take the child away. We're not doing it anymore because it's not worth it". You start to . . .'. Mike constructs himself as so powerless that he considers behaviours that he does not wish to use. This resonates with Brian's efforts to access services for different children and finding himself in conflict with the department:

> [Y]ou're really powerless . . . Sometimes I've got really angry and I've had numerous rows with social workers. But it's not always easy . . . usually we've always ended up sorting it out amicably but sometimes it's had to be after a few pretty terse words.

Foster carers feel that they know intimately the care needs of the children but when social services fail to respond, then feelings of powerlessness lead to anger. Regularly the foster carers construct their fostering lives as without autonomy in relation to the local authority. They describe the social services as being in control. This control, demonstrated through surveillance and criticism, can be personal. Miranda, an experienced childminder but newly registered foster carer, describes herself as 'devastated' when, having been advised in a child-care lecture to use 'time-out'[2] with children, found that it was an issue with her Family Placement social worker. Members of the Foster Care Panel visited her for discussion and, 'it still hurts me now . . . I'm sure it depends on which social worker you're talking to'.

Miranda experiences the uncertainties which arise from differing expectations. More than her authority, her sense of worth and her identity have been undermined. She places this within the context of the idiosyncratic power of the local authority and its ability to intrude upon personal child-care choices and practice. There are many examples of what could be regarded as intrusion into the personal choices and lives of foster carers. Dick and his cousin Simon live with Dick's mother. The three of them applied to foster but Dick found:

> [W]e did have an awful lot of trouble actually getting approved . . .
> I lived with a partner for some years but never married, which gave me
> a lot of this come-back that, we was gay . . . what he [Family Placement
> social worker] was saying was the chap that's a Chairman of the Panel
> doesn't get on with him, so there's a little bit of friction there.

Dick had to give his social worker a list of past girl-friends; 'it was like the
Spanish Inquisition actually'. All local authorities are supposed to have an
equal opportunities policy which covers the selection of foster carers and
allows for applicants from the gay community. In this case the cousins say
they are heterosexual and are obliged to prove this, apparently because
there is some friction between their assessor and a member of the Fostering
Panel. Dick did not resist this examination of his sexuality. It is as though,
sometimes, foster carers see themselves, and feel themselves, to be so powerless in the face of the local authority that they actively co-operate with
actions which are unjust and unreasonable. Apparently unquestioningly
Dick gave his social worker names and addresses. These actions positively
manufacture the power of the social care department.

Carers indicate that they mistrust the local authority's power and are wary
of the department's decisions. Yvonne, although requesting registration for
three teenagers, was granted two until a crisis resulted in the department
persuading her to use her dining room for an extra boy, 'so that was the
bedroom. Then another boy came in and used that as a bedroom and
another *girl* came . . . And *now* I've been passed by Social Services as I've
got three . . . They've passed it to suit themselves'.

The interviews indicate that frequently foster carers relinquish personal
agency in the face of social services' demands. Their sense of powerlessness,
of otherness, means that they allow social workers to take decisions which
affect their private, personal lives. This is illustrated by social services' attitude to 'Safer Caring' practices. Olivia tells how one teenage girl constantly
ran away and, when found, Isambard had to collect her; the male social
worker refusing to escort her in line with Safer Caring procedures.

Stan recalls social workers bringing a small girl to his house, when Laura
was out. The child was filthy and the social workers reported that they
suspected that she had been sexually abused and requested that he bath her.
They neither offered to do this themselves nor remained to chaperone.
Bureaucratic care provides rules and regulations but not practical solutions.
Foster carers are left to grapple with the pragmatic realities which may
affect, in their perception, the quality of their care.

Several carers describe how social services discriminate in favour of foster
children against birth children. They relate incidents where departmental
insistence of the foster child's paramountcy reduces the status of the birth
children to second place. Alice's social worker telephones daily to inquire
about the fostered toddler but not how Alice's young and jealous daughter

is coping.[3] Louise, with an ill daughter, talks of the priority given to the foster baby, Victoria:

> [A]ll I wanted to do was get Emily to the doctors . . . so I phoned up and said 'I can't do it' [Victoria's contact] and I explained why, and I had a stroppy letter, 'you signed an agreement to say that you didn't mind contact every day at your house' and we actually had a meeting which took place here and the social worker . . . went to say 'well we have had problems when Louise got on her high horse', and I said 'well excuse me I do get on my high horse, I've got a daughter with a temperature of one hundred and two, who has febrile convulsions. My priority was my daughter and not my foster child' . . . but my kids aren't allowed to be ill.

Foster carers who believe that they are selected for their parenting skills suggest that they are pressured into letting their standards slip with regard to their birth children. In general parents accept responsibility for their own children. But there is a subtle demand to ensure that care for the foster children takes precedence. It is a dilemma. Louise is obliged to reconstruct her notions of conscientious standards of care and must now finely balance the needs of the foster child with her own three. There is a moral responsibility to put children's needs first, but not all children are regarded as equal.

All family members are affected by fostering. Ruth is explicit: 'It was me and my two children and *we* cared. *We* were foster carers . . . They didn't take any of the parental rights but they still had the babysitting to do, the "will you just mind this while I just go do this?"' Foster care can generate an expectation of more adult behaviours; birth children may get constructed as more understanding and more able/useful.

Ali Shah bemoans the unsought-for changes within his household:

> [I]f a [foster] child is in our family he will not be treated any differently *unless* the system force us. Otherwise we will give them *every* way like we give our own . . . [but] you have to tell your [own] children, 'Behave differently with your foster children' . . . When they fight you call both of them . . . tell them off and say go away. Now you can't do this with a foster child. You see foster child will always come to you and he will want proper answers. He would say '*Why?*' Now your child cannot say that to the parents, 'Why?' You always tell them to get lost or shut up or something, and you can't say this to a foster child. You have to explain all the time. For *that* you have to tell your children not to go that far so we'll have to explain everything.

Accepting its clear cultural implications, nonetheless this extract illustrates other carers' complaints, the clash of expectations regarding their ideas of parental authority and that of the social services. Whilst carers may believe that foster children deserve better/more, this is supported by departmental practice and underpinned by children's rights. Hanneke's view is that this is impractical. Describing life with one child:

> [S]he says 'you're not allowed to touch me . . . you try and restrain me and *I* will say something else' . . . the Social *Worker* will *always* take *her* side . . . So if you can't touch them . . . you can't restrain them, you can't do anything, it's impossible really . . . Now they've got all the power . . . She would torment my four-year-old with a stick. You'd call her in and before you even opened your mouth she says, 'It's not fair', screams, bawls . . . slump onto the floor . . . she'll say, 'You're not allowed to touch me. I'm going to go the social services. I'm going to tell'. Now when the other children, obviously looking on, they see this behaviour and they learn what? How I'm incapable of doing anything and think 'Well *I* can get away with it. *She* can get away with it'.

These extracts demonstrate how the social services' efforts at ensuring the protection of foster children's rights can have unintended consequences. As carers feel disempowered the foster children are thereby constructed as powerful.

Foster carers also construct the birth parents of the children as powerful. Local authorities have a legal duty to promote family contact and parents retain, or at least share, parental responsibility which gives them rights to be consulted with regard to their children. This study confirms Cleaver's findings (2000) that the children's birth families become a real part of foster family life. Mandy, Harry and Miranda complain of the inconvenience caused by contact arrangements in their homes. Louise, with three daughters, has to retire to a bedroom for an hour each day whilst social services supervise family visits downstairs. Although finding this onerous, like other foster carers, she gives priority to the child's needs. Hanneke's experience of respite care is that parents visit beforehand to 'check her out'. She accepts this, believing her task to be that of working and complying with their requests. She speaks of their 'rights' and constructs birth parents as having, in this context, more rights than herself. In this case 'rights' equate to power and some control.

Olivia's baby is visited daily by her mother who refuses the offer of lunch so the family cannot eat until after two o'clock. The mother complains that her son is frightened of Olivia's daughter, who is a child with Down syndrome, so Olivia takes her out. The understanding of these carers is that parental wishes and local authority child-care philosophy takes precedence over their positions as foster carers, even within their homes. Their perception is that the birth parents hold the power and the rights whilst they, the carers, have the responsibilities.

The general response to the hypothetical vignette regarding a child's contact with an alcoholic father at the same time as a family party was an insistence upon the importance of contact, with ten carers offering to include the parents at their own family function. These ten perceived their own arrangements as subservient to those of the child and her birth family. In discussion, individuals related occasions when they had, at great personal inconvenience, honoured contact arrangements. Many carers talk sympathetically of the birth families. Ruth includes in her account of a typical day, counselling her foster child's mother. Laura receives Mothers Day cards from mothers in recognition of her support. Each evening, on the telephone, Mary reassures a birth mother that she is not displacing her maternal role in the child's affections. Khanm Shah regularly offers meals.

However, relationships between birth parents and foster carers can be fickle. Tricia fostered baby Josh for ten months until his death. He visited his grandparents each weekend, though if there was a health problem they summoned Tricia, 'I *thought* we had a good relationship'. When it was clear that he was ill Tricia took him to hospital,

> we knew he wouldn't live and so I got Granny up there . . . and, bless him, he died. And she said, 'You can go . . . *This* will be our *private* business now' . . . all through his other illnesses I'd done all the dirty bits. She'd just had some nice cuddling care really and they *never* invited us to his funeral.

Tricia had constructed her foster carer role as central to Josh's life only to find that his birth family regarded her as peripheral and expendable and could assert their boundaries.

There are other difficulties. Hanneke and Isambard cope with birth parents who wish to remove children. If Laura is out, Stan asks neighbours to act as chaperones when young mothers visit wearing 'pelmets'. Harold knows a foster carer who was rammed by a birth parent's car. There is some resistance to parents' demands and behaviours. Grace, for example, requests the removal of a child because his mother's aggressive telephone calls frighten her daughter. But Laura still sees a mother who arrived at midnight and broke a window to gain entry. The social services' response is that their insurance covers damage done by the foster children, but not by their parents.

Although incidents are recounted as unfair, there is no real sense of grievance from these carers. In their descriptions it is clear that they are living with these difficulties rather than consciously reflecting upon them. Ruth refers to anything that she perceives as negative in foster care as 'her lot'. It is as if carers construct themselves as victims and present foster care as a package which inevitably includes hardship and injustice in return for the care of the children.

Generally the study carers talked of wanting 'to make a difference to some children's lives' (Emma). They clearly anticipate this 'difference' in positive terms because, as Mo asserts, 'those people who know Lindsey, they know the difference'. Alice reports that the social worker describes her fostered toddler as 'a totally different person'. Thus implicit in 'making the difference' is an intention to make better and to reverse some sort of damage caused by earlier experiences; to rescue spoiled or harmed children as Daisy illustrates:

> Seeing what the problem is and try and help them . . . to try and make that bad child better or a happier child . . . I think like a good happy family, a nice home, nice comfortable rooms for the child you know just that family *unit* thing really, including the child in everything and making them feel part of your family, which I think that, that child really needs . . . they need that love and care, they need security more than anything and I think routine is wonderful for children . . . knowing there is normal life there.

Daisy's construction of foster care is dependent upon some of our understandings of family. As explored earlier, sociology literature identifies 'family' as an ideological concept; a social unit offering internal cohesion with external boundaries. Family offers a shared residential basis with a fundamental division between adults and children, encouraging care, nurture and team effort, with an equitable distribution of resources within hierarchical divisions and around age categories. There are strong orientations to time past and to the future, with traditions and a shared history. Importantly there is a set of taken-for-granted assumptions about how 'family' operates; it is all effortless and natural. The 'naturalness' may be a product of biology or sentiment, but it is outside of law, contract, or self-interest.[4] Daisy's description has elements of this idealism; foster carers can 'make a bad child better' by the provision of family and home and a 'normal life'. She envisages rescuing children with love and care and routine; by 'doing' family.

Kelly, an experienced carer, reflects:

> I was hoping to give what they'd missed out on. But I actually feel that's impossible . . . You can't replace their natural family. You can't undo the damage that they've experienced . . . I just wanted to be able to give to children, which I still do, and try and give them as normal a life as possible in a family . . . a fresh start. You know we wanted to try and bring him up in a family that was *normal*.

Whilst recognising the impossibility of repairing children's lives, Kelly nonetheless constructs herself and her husband as a 'normal' family who can provide the foster children with new opportunities. Some idealism remains as she promotes the view that they can rescue children for 'a fresh start'.

Integral rescue ingredients for both of these carers are notions of 'home' and 'family'. Both are certain that there is a common, comprehensible definition of both which equates to 'normal'. Neither of these carers have birth children so it could be argued that the foster children offer them 'family' rather than vice versa. Kelly, responding to the first vignette on page 118 (pressurising a foster family to take an extra girl), decides, 'You've got to put your own family first'.

Others demonstrate this same adamant regard for the significance of family. Yvonne includes foster children '*in* the family circle'. Laura expounds her construction of family and home:

> I believe in children eating all together, you know, *as a family* . . . You're just a normal family . . . a home where they come in, they go to the fridge, shoes are there, which they are, and coats. I mean some nights the house is, you know, with coats here, chucked there, the bedrooms are a mess but, why should everything be put in its place? . . . that's not *home* for children. I don't think.

Laura's construction of family maps onto her notion of home. It requires a space where children feel free, unrestricted, uncriticised and share meals.[5] This unconditional acceptance contrasts with Ali Shah; his concern is actively teaching children to adopt (his) acceptable manners and ways of behaviour. Something of this is reflected in Frances' construction of fostering:

> I just feel so much that a good family gives so much stability to an individual and if we can be involved in any way in helping to give confidence or, stability, to young people that's really what I hope that we can achieve.

Her wish to instil stability and confidence into young people is heavily predicated upon her notion of providing 'a good family'. It is this which comprises the rescue package. Georgina, experiencing full-time employment as incompatible with foster care, describes her 'ideal' foster family as:

> [B]eing able to give them a warm house to live in and a family . . . she [foster carer] can spend all day with them and they all play together and that's the ideal family. Then she takes them on trips and has got all the time in the world for them.

Home bestows personal fulfilment but maintaining the idea of home requires a continuous effort at ensuring collective activities (Kumar, 1997). Georgina's construction rests upon the full-time mother figure spending her time playing with the children[6] and taking them on trips. It is these activities that construct both the family and the model site for fostering. Warmth commences as the physical (the house/home) and becomes the emotional, the ideal family.

Family is about a sense of identity, belonging and intimacy. Although offering a 'family' some carers struggle with describing this complex construction. Kelly states 'in our house none of us are related', whilst Ann says her two boys (in touch with their parents who have very different social mores) are 'not us'; blood ties are omnipotent and social behaviours count. Ruth is clear that:

> We try to work as a family, but I don't call it a *family*. I say this *house*. . . . They *have* a family. They don't *need* another family . . . What they need is a safe place to be, somewhere where they know they are cared for and loved and looked after . . . So this is what it is. It's my house, their home.

Ruth's foster children have birth families so do not need her to replicate and substitute another. She may not refer to her household as 'family' although that is how it operates as she reproduces this notion by offering her 'house (as) their home'. This extract demonstrates the complexities of the foster carers' worlds; how their efforts to care for the children entail continuously positioning and repositioning themselves in order to 'make a difference' or to 'make the children's lives better'.

Rescuing children and making a difference is about change. All the foster carers reflect on this in their interviews. For most this is their raison d'être as they believe that their influence, intervention and contribution can beneficially change the lives of children; they want to give the foster children the benefit of a 'proper childhood'. As Mary articulates, 'You know you can't give everything, even if it was your own child, and so you realise "I can do something different"'. For Grace the delight in fostering is: '[T]o see the *change* in the children. When they come they're so distracted . . . so upset. They don't know what to think . . . And then to see a change, is like a magic and they *change*.' Grace's care of foster children produces such dramatic alteration that she likens it to magic. Mary constructs what happens to the children as something which is personal to herself and the result of her own power to transform and to make a difference. Dick details this with regard to Derrick:

> He's 16 going on 12 . . . this is the only one I really feel that I'm actually fostering because he does need help learning everything . . . he will listen to you and you can see that he takes notice of what you say and he comes to you for advice.

Dick's construction of himself as foster carer is that change is required for Derrick and that he, Dick, is the agent. For the first time he knows himself to be instrumental so that he is now, with this lad, reassured that he is actually fostering; actively making a difference. For Dick life-as-foster-carer is life-as-change-agent.

Although all the carers talked about the importance of change, it can be uncertain.

> Rewards are very delayed. Sometimes the disappointments are that you never get to see whether or not you've had an effect, but the rewards are when you know you have . . . For example, taking a child in who'd been excluded from school . . . and by the time he left you he was back in mainstream school.
>
> (Isambard)

Change only has a magic for some if they experience and witness it, although Hanneke is more pragmatic and suggests a long-term view:

> I want my [birth] children not to be a burden on anybody. I want them to make sure that they can look after themselves and if you can help another child do the same it will save all those, I won't say crimes . . . trying to do the preventative thing, actually looking ahead.

Foster carers only know if their care has been adequate/produced the required change by following progress. But Hanneke views childhood as a process, a developing career, and herself-as-foster-carer able to influence this in some way for the better. The parent–child relationship functions on a foundation that childhood is a continuing changing state and Hanneke appreciates the long-term meaningfulness of motherhood. The child embodies their own future and, with this in mind, Hanneke constructs herself as foster-carer-as-change-agent.

Foster-carer-as-change-agent can ameliorate negative situations. Stuart, recollecting a child whose behaviour he considered so damaging to his family that he requested her removal recalls, 'her school work changed hugely so we know one success . . . From being the most terrible difficult child she did tremendously well'. Change can gratify and compensate. This is important because, as other quotations demonstrate, life-as-foster-carer can be distressingly difficult. So should foster carers be recompensed?

The majority of foster carers in this country are unpaid; they care for children in return for an allowance which does not meet the costs (Oldfield, 1997). Zelizer (1985) posits that allowances never cover the expenditure since it is the non-economic part of the contract that legitimises the scheme; the emotional attachment must be more than the financial connection.

In this study, 23 foster households are in receipt of allowances only. The other four (Meg, Lenin, Clive and Kelly, Mike and Louise) are on special schemes whereby each household receives the allowance(s) plus an additional fee. Harry, Brian and Mike explain that fostering fits their life-style as their wives are at home anyway. Children can offer women a retreat from the working world and some may foster in order to demonstrate that their husbands keep them; of the 14 work-age index couples, 6 wives have paid occupations, 3 of them full time.

The majority of the study carers constantly distance themselves from allowances and payments. It is as though they believe that money under-mines their care status. Nonetheless all of them have views on the fiscal arrangements and the ambiguities of caring for money, so finance clearly impacts upon foster carer identities. In general there is a weariness about the fact that the social care services are not straightforward about the costs of fostering. The allowance scales are known but not which extra expenses can be claimed. This extract from Ruth's interview regarding payment is typical:

> I *hate* talking about it . . . because that's not what I'm *here* to do . . . I'm not doing it to make money . . . I mean it's *not* a living. Being a single parent you see, we were very limited, financially. And in the very, very beginning it was very, very difficult to meet all these demands that were made upon us. To see to these children socially, to see to their fun, to see to their clothing, you know, because 90 per cent of these children came without clothes and to *have* to get on the phone and prac-tically *beg* for money was, not humiliating for me but humiliating for these children, specially if they heard me . . .
>
> And I had to struggle to buy a car. Nobody came forward and said, 'Now you've learnt to drive and you're going to take the children here, there and everywhere, do you want us to insure the car or, you know, sort of buy the road tax for you?' I didn't want them to *buy* the car . . . but perhaps they could have helped in other little ways. I mean it's *their* children that I ferry backwards and forwards.

For Ruth, money and care are distinct issues but, dependent upon state benefits, she is reliant upon the fostering allowances to care for public children. She finds this problematic. For her, financial discussion is an embarrassment; she does not construct her requests as entitlement but rather as a supplication. Elsewhere she explains that the car is essentially for the foster children, but does not feel reciprocally supported by the local authority.

Leat's work (1990) establishes that although foster carers do not look after children for money, they do feel that caring, without payment, should not be expected. Sinclair and colleagues (2004) note that the quality of care is affected by poor financial support. Although aligning herself with these per-spectives, Ruth, in common with most study foster carers, constructs caring as distinct from, if not superior to, finance. Dealing with the practicalities of foster care costs is difficult and painful.

Reconciling care and payment can be a struggle for some foster carers as 'work is love made visible' (Gibran, 1923: 38). Ruth constructs life-as-unpaid-foster-carer as separate from money since families, 'are, distinctively, places within which the common currency of money, of profit, of loss, of "rational" economic exchange, is out of place' (Hood-Williams, 1990: 159). Thus she, like others, is careful to explain that she does not look after children for payment. Stan states, 'I don't think you can put a price on a child's head'. Children are priceless; their value is above cost. Wakeford (1963) suggests that foster children fulfil a social rather than an economic role; middle-class women find alternative goals within the home but working-class women need another child, or at least a child, to give significance to their lives.

Several talk of fostering being a 'job' or a 'business' in the same way as some women describe full-time mothering. Richard's extract illustrates many of their statements and constructions:

> You're part of a business . . . and it is a job 'cos you get paid for it . . . you're the carer for the kids . . . you get an allowance . . . so technically you're paid for it and you know it's not enough . . .
>
> I've been saying about the money and it sounds like that's the most important thing, but it isn't . . . we just happened to have placements which cost an arm and a leg to kit them out from day one . . . It cost her [Mary, his wife] an arm and a leg looking after these, it's silly things like the amount of time, the washing and ironing and that sort of stuff, it's ludicrous, but I wouldn't say, if you said to me would I change it? No, I would say, I'm quite happy doing it.

Richard is self-employed so this extract illustrates the contradictions and complexities concerning payment for foster carers. His own time is costed out yet in fostering his wife gives her time for free. Even though he can see the inconsistency he states that he will continue to foster. Yet because they are in receipt of (only) allowances, Richard's instinctive metaphor for foster care is that of a business. He constructs Mary's fostering as part of the local authority's formal care of children; it is foster-care-as-unwaged-work.

Similar conundrums concerning payment are voiced regularly in this study. Purchasing love is morally unacceptable; it must be freely given but the principle of payment is important. Miranda strives to reconcile payment for care:

> It's difficult . . . you don't want to attract people to fostering for the wrong reasons . . . I need the money and sometimes I feel bad about that . . . am I doing it for the wrong reasons? 'Cos if I wasn't paid I wouldn't do it. I wouldn't do it because I'm only doing it because I want the money, but I wouldn't do it because I couldn't physically afford to.

Even though, without an allowance, she cannot afford to foster, Miranda expresses guilt about the financial arrangements. Several foster carers find problematic the receipt/reimbursement of monies and therefore justify the transactions. Yvonne, for example, lists the number of television sets in the house and how much food she purchases each week. For many foster carers the construction of foster-carer-in-receipt-of-money proves uncomfortable. This includes Mike whose wife fosters for a fee:

> Victoria [foster child] gets an allowance which isn't a lot . . . I mean it's for the work that Louise does. It's a 24-hour-a-day job . . . I think it's more of a, an acknowledgement payment I think. I mean you certainly wouldn't go into this for financial gain by any means . . . I've said to him [Family Placement social worker] how can you sift through the people that are doing it purely for financial reasons when people like us want to do it to help?

For Mike fostering is not a business but an activity that suits his family. But the fact of Louise's fee does not fit comfortably with his notion of genuine, wanting-to-do-it care. He needs to ensure that people understand the difference; that they want to foster anyway. For him any construction of foster-carer-as-paid-agent must clarify that they are not doing it for the money. This is a stance mirrored by Lenin, also fee paid, who 'never went into it for the money'. Because she receives a fee, Kelly will not ask her mother to babysit; she and Clive go out on separate evenings. Thus foster-carer-as-paid-agent is constructed by her as the local authority purchasing 24-hour care and complete accountability.

However, there are variations. Meg, also fee paid, is comfortable with an instrumental construction of foster-carer-as-paid-agent. She describes her adolescent lads as expensive and hard work. Hanneke feels strongly that all foster carers should be paid:

> I mean the trauma that you go through both emotionally and physically having to deal with them, I think *more* than just *expenses* should be paid . . . it's like a nurse you know. I mean doing it for nothing is hard going and probably less likely for it to be successful because you think, well what am I doing this for? This child doesn't seem to want our care. Why should I care? . . . We do a 'job' and we should be fairly paid . . . we should not have to subsidise the foster children. As things are at the moment we are happy to give of our time and our caring and love, but not the money as well.

Tricia, fostering children with multiple disabilities, argues along similar lines:

> I do just feel quite strongly that in lots of situations we are *not* listened to or recognised for what we're doing, what we're offering. The *commitment*

that we're offering . . . the recognition is *not* always there . . . with disabilities . . . you're going to get basic [allowances] and I'm afraid I
don't agree with that for nursing care, not 24-hour nursing care. It's
just not on . . . we're not looking for a great fee . . . But I just think something should be there.

Both carers state that they already give the local authority more than the
allowances justify. Hanneke's construction of her fostering is that the local
authority can expect to have her time, her caring and her love for the
children for free but that there should be compensatory payments for the
frustrations and the emotional and physical exhaustion. She constructs
fostering as a job, as (un)paid work. Moreover, foster-carer-as-paid-agent
she constructs as warranting more accountability in order to confirm success
in difficult placements; a fee would purchase even more effort. Tricia has
fostered three children with terminal illnesses. The current baby requires
tube-feeding, regular resuscitation and general nursing. Yet none of this
effort or experience is recognised and she wants financial acknowledgement,
however minor. For both these carers, foster-carer-as-paid-agent is constructed as the local council recognising and rewarding the fact that foster
carers regularly do more than is realised. Overall there is a sense of financial
exploitation; foster carers expect to give love but feel aggrieved that others
take advantage.

Many of the study foster carers appear to be subsidising the children.
Gordon and Emma keep the children out of their salaries and use the allowances for clothes, toys and outings. Mike complains that Victoria regularly
requires new clothing and that this is purchased from his wife's fee. Laura
remembers the arrival of a new foster child the day before a family wedding:
'I went out that Friday and I bought her clothes to go to this wedding. I can
remember as if it was yesterday, it was our mortgage money'.

Some carers, like Hanneke and Tricia do not see fostering as incompatible
with payment, but together with Meg and Mike, who also construct foster-
carers-as-paid-agents, they are in the minority.[7] Many of them, although
expressing dissatisfaction with the financial arrangements, nonetheless
agree with Brian:

I sometimes think we must be mad and I sometimes say to Tricia, 'I just
don't know *why* you just don't go out and get yourself a job, nine to five
and, you know, we'll know *exactly* where we are, we know when we can
take holidays . . . what our life structure will be and everything else'.
But we always go back to the same thing, *it's not what we want to do.*
You know, fostering is what we want to do.

Understanding why foster carers 'want' to foster is complex and examined in
other literature but this study confirms one source of motivation. Ten carers
had either parents who fostered, or had been in the care system themselves.

Hanneke's grandparents and parents had looked after children so she feels that fostering is a natural life event. This is true for Margaret and Dick. Georgina's mother fostered, as did Miranda's, though Miranda's reason is couched in emotionality:

> One of the *biggest things that made me want to do it* was when I was 17 we fostered this girl . . . probably for two or three weeks . . . she started sending Christmas cards every year to my mum and then when my mum died she turned up at the funeral with a big bunch of flowers and it, oh it just chokes me up just thinking about it, but what my mum did for that girl in three weeks had such an impression on her that five, six, seven years later she would take a bunch of flowers to her funeral and that really made me want to foster 'cos I thought if she could do that for somebody then I'd like to do that too.

Elsewhere in interview Miranda explains that her decision to foster is because she wants more children but the inspiration is this experience. For her, life-as-foster-carer is also about homage to her mother and an ambition to give the same meaningful experience to another child. Some of this resonates with Stuart's account. Orphaned at the age of 12 arrangements were made for him to live with a local family. He refers to this couple as his foster parents and enjoyed a close relationship with his foster father, so that now:

> We have one who has taken *me* to his heart in the same way that I took *my* foster father to his [sic] heart . . .
>   He enjoys being with me, I enjoy being with him. I'm *his* sort of person and he's *my* sort of person . . . He rushes in, 'Stuart I want to see you' . . . I'm looking forward to my weekend, I really look *forward* to my weekends.

Stuart, like Miranda, takes a meaningful experience from his past and strives to replicate it. In the same way that he models himself upon his foster father he is now delighted to foster at weekends a boy whom he perceives to be fond of him. For these two individuals their construction of foster carer includes reworking a positive role from their childhood. Jackie's account is similar as she makes connections from her own fostering model. She describes her years in foster care as: 'a very positive experience . . . I still keep in contact with the family . . . I learnt the caring, setting the *standards* from them'.

Foster care, for these last three, is about replicative scripts and long-term time orientations and continuity. But for Laura, who was in a children's home and Gordon, who was fostered, foster care is about corrective scripts ensuring discontinuity and changing the life course. Gordon explains:

I was treated very badly . . . they abused me . . . the main thing was, there was mental abuse. They would say things to me and promise me things and threaten me with things . . . They made me play in a shed three feet by three feet with no door in it in the middle of winter and with short trousers on and a, [near to tears] and a shirt, freezing cold. I used to have porridge for my breakfast, a sandwich for my dinner and porridge for my tea, it was really bad . . . I can reverse that. Couldn't I? I can give somebody a good life.

It is important to Gordon to give children a contrasting experience from his own.[8] He wants to reverse his treatment so his construction of foster care includes physical and emotional warmth, security and reassurance. He wants to take his own negative experience of abuse and offer children a positive time. Being a foster carer is, for Gordon, about ensuring difference.

But if and when they make any difference, how responsible do the foster carers feel for the children? Examination of the transcripts provides general conformity. Most of the carers in response to the vignette about bullying accept responsibility for the foster child and wish to persevere with the placement. Though some, like Meg, are more pragmatic, matter-of-fact about those who do not flourish whilst proud of those who do. Remembering Roger she says:

I felt as if I'd done a *really good* success story over that boy because he was a boy that literally *everyone* . . . *everyone* foresaid he would spend the rest of his life on the dole, on the scrap heap, no one would want him. He's been in the same job, he's 21 this year . . . So we both proved everybody wrong! I feel quite good about it, Roger, actually.

In a proprietorial parental way, Meg is claiming that some of Roger's success is because of herself, enough for her to own some pride in him. Although she does not talk about failing with other teenagers (Wes's continual conflicts with the law or her current lad's inability to settle) nonetheless, in some circumstances she, like a parent, constructs foster care as including responsibility for outcomes for children, albeit selected ones.

Stan and Laura struggle with this same construction. New carers telephone them for advice. Stan explains, 'people must understand that they are not a failure if the first placement isn't successful . . . they mustn't be, feel they've failed'. Laura agrees:

New foster parents ring up and say, you know, 'I can't handle this you know, we're a failure'. I say *'no you're not a failure* just 'cos you can't keep the first ones'. . . . I felt that with, the one that we, that was very close to my son [a foster girl who fell in love with Laura's son], you know, we kept for eight months and then realised . . . it was *our son's home* and not her permanent home. So we had to give her up but it wasn't so much that it was, oh I don't know, I don't you know, it's ever so difficult, it's really, you know.

Here Laura struggles but cannot state that, in requesting the removal of a foster child, she has not failed. She can advise new carers to believe this but knows how she feels. Implicitly she constructs foster care as taking responsibility for children's futures. Elsewhere she explains how the girl's behaviour made life impossible for her son and led to the disruption of the placement. Nonetheless Laura does not here put the responsibility back onto the girl, but struggles with where to place it. Parents can be held to account for their children; their moral identity is bound up with behaviour and Laura feels morally accountable for children who are not hers.

This same accountability is also evident when strangers frequently assume that foster children are blood children. Hanneke, describing life with one child, explains the absence of family outings as the child was prone to tantrums and Hanneke feared the (unspoken) criticism of other adults. Although not accepting responsibility for the child's behaviour, Hanneke believes that other people would consider her liable. Adults are held accountable for the actions of children in their care. Since they have had Dylan, Georgina has not visited her great aunt 'because I dread to think if he broke something'. Her construction of foster care is that she accepts that, like parents, they are held publicly responsible for children's (unacceptable) behaviour. Similarly Celia is aware of public scrutiny where her control of foster children is concerned. She does not want, 'people to point their finger and say, "Well look. She's looking after this child and she can't control this child . . . What useless parents"'. Mandy is relieved to witness other children's tantrums and notes, 'well Timmy is better than them, I don't think I have to apologise for anything . . . *we are doing very well*'.

Generally mothers in contemporary Western societies feel socially accountable for their children's behaviour (Ribbens, 1994; Ruddick, 1983). So foster carers, like parents, compare quite competitively children's conduct and manners. Mandy's construction of foster care includes responsibility for general behaviour and pride in behaviour which is acceptable. But many of these carers, particularly the experienced carers, speak of feeling disheartened when accepting (voluntarily) responsibility for disappointments with children. Although acknowledging that the children present exceptionally difficult behaviours, they nonetheless talk of their own failings, as exemplified by Kelly:

Roy is a particularly disturbed child with such extreme behaviour . . . he actually set fire to a teacher's hair and threatened another member of staff with scissors . . . he's injured one of our dogs. I think we've done the right thing [agreeing to his removal] . . . I still keep in touch with him . . . We get jobs, we get married, we have a family . . . I can't see any of that going well for him and I feel very, very sad about that and I always will do and I don't think I will ever get over that. It damaged my confidence a lot because I felt really confident with the success of Jane and then Nathan. I felt great! . . . I know we've had a failure with Roy, in my opinion it was a failure.

Kelly accepts responsibility for success and for failure. She knows that Roy's behaviour is dangerous yet continues to question herself. For Kelly the foster carer is constructed as responsible for the children; their behaviour and their future lives.

Similarly Dick remembers how Jamie was told (erroneously) that he could remain with him but was then moved. In his outrage Jamie held the foster family at knifepoint for several hours:

I feel a total failure with him because he, every week he's at the Police Station getting had up for something or other, but you know I mean, I tend to blame myself but it's not my fault, it's that social worker's fault, but you know what I mean.

Dick states that it was not his actions that led to the disruption of the place-ment and Jamie's subsequent decline into offending. Nevertheless, like Kelly and many others, he constructs foster carers as people who must rescue and save young people. When this is not possible it is regarded as a personal failure which cannot be discounted and forgotten. Jackie muses over the youngsters who are not managing their lives successfully, 'you always think back and think to yourself, could I have done something different with that relationship?' Any success or failure is constructed with great intimacy; it is the carer's personality at stake. The foster carers' sense of care is about connectedness; they can be so intimately bound up with others that they invite the burden.

Celia's sister accompanied them on a holiday which was wrecked by the behaviour of a foster child:

But even then when we came off holiday she didn't actually say, 'Because it was your [Celia's] fault, but you ruined our holiday'. You know. And her holiday *was* ruined, through me . . . All I can think of was the fact that it was all too much for him because in his family life he was never taken anywhere.

Celia's belief, like other study carers, that children cannot be blamed means that she takes responsibility for their behaviour. This particular construction means that explanation for unacceptable conduct does not exonerate the carer.

But, like Meg and Kelly, carers also take credit for successes. Stan is delighted that Stacey is at college 'and come on really well'. Kathleen's pride in Ruby means that she insists that they sit together in church, 'so more of the congregation would have realised that, that was our little girl, but up until that point we were not able to show her off'. As with all children, foster children are called upon for display purposes and for companionship (Hood-Williams, 1990). Like Cyril, who wants his friends to approve of Craig, and Grace who 'suit(s) them all out', Kathleen is concerned about the public presentation of her foster child. But additionally some study carers construct themselves as taking full responsibility for their foster children: for their physical appearance, their public behaviours and their (future) personal happiness, whatever their status within the family.

Expectations about fairness in family life demand that fostered children receive parity with birth children although social services' expectations may be that their interests be prioritised. This chapter has explored some of the carers' constructions of their status with regard to the social care departments, the birth parents and the foster children. Foster carers present themselves as often powerless; their authority and their boundaries heavily compromised as they must always be mindful of the children's birth families, children's rights and the ever-present local council. Foster carers lack both legal power and authority. The birth parents have legal power whilst the social services department have authority.

Organisations, and in this case the social care departments, provide routine ways of representing social reality. Foster carers are part of the social service bureaucracy but their place is unclear and ambiguous. The bureaucracy and its staff have apparent roles and legally based powers. The foster children and their parents have specified rights. Foster carers have none of these but must somehow construct their roles and shape their lives in ways that allow them to navigate through all these complexities. Their attitudes towards the social service departments are ambiguous and paradoxical. This chapter has noted their frustrations and their hurts at bureaucracy's inability to appreciate the detail of care required for each individual child. Yet, at the same time, carers enjoy the visits of the social workers, they appreciate inclusion at meetings and experience kudos from the many 'business' telephone calls and appointments.

Foster carers do not only offer the provision of physical shelter and care but also an emotional, expressive relationship which is sometimes made problematic by the payment of monies. Generally they construct themselves as intimately connected to the children. This purposeful particularistic tie enables them to act as change agents for the children and to rescue them from their pasts. Theirs is a powerful account of the management of behaviour. Fostering is about making things better for the children; changing children must therefore be personally gratifying for the carers.

5 Having a presence through children

Although the foster carers were not specifically asked during interviews about the children, previous chapters have indicated their centrality. The analysis will therefore now shift the focus onto children-within-foster-families in order to consider how the carers construct them and whether this is in a particular way. This requires an initial discussion of some of the literature considering the construction of childhood.

Whilst the debate continues as to whether the contemporary Western construction of childhood is extending or disappearing (Jenks, 1996), there is general literary agreement about its social construction. Fundamentally, categories of child and adult are seen as separate (Pilcher, 1995) because of their differences from each other, and childhood itself has been institutionalised and depicted in particular terms. It is seen as a separate stage/state/concept during the life course (Hendrick, 1990). This is demonstrated in the ideology around the special site of 'home' as the most appropriate place for children, in the legislation for their full-time education and exclusion from the labour market, and in the demarcation of particular places, e.g. play parks, specifically for their use. Parallel to this theme of separateness is an emphasis on children's incompetence, vulnerability and dependence (Boyden, 1990). Childhood is constructed as a time for children to benefit and to enjoy. Ribbens McCarthy and colleagues' review of the literature (2000) concludes that contemporary opinion agrees that the child is constructed as innocent; children are not expected to be responsible since care-taking adults are morally accountable for their actions. Thus children are, by contrast, 'non-persons' and the ideology of childhood, positioning the child as innocent and not accountable, maps onto macro notions of power and the child's relatively powerless position. This in itself reinforces the polarisation of a morally accountable adult and the construction of the child as without moral agency, whose needs are seen as paramount.

Zelizer (1985) explores the change from the past position of the child, as an economic family unit, to today's economically worthless child perceived as an expensive and emotionally priceless sentimental asset. She links this to the domestication, and redefining, of middle-class women in the nineteenth century paralleling the new concept of the child as so precious as to be sacrilised. In return for this status contemporary Western children are expected to provide love, smiles and emotional satisfaction. It is the total enchantment of childhood (Beck and Beck-Gernsheim, 1995; Zelizer, 1985). Couples have children for non-monetary benefits; children have sentimental value as parents desire love and affection and the feeling of being a family (ibid.). Children are perceived as a claim to happiness; they make life meaningful (Beck and Beck-Gernsheim, 1995).

In general terms the contemporary Western child is constructed as so innocent and so priceless that their needs are supreme. Childhood demands as of right adult labour, expensive goods and an intense emotional involvement (Jenks, 1994). This construction is central to the accounts of the foster carers in the study. But as this chapter will demonstrate they construct their foster children as not only 'priceless' but, because they are bureaucratised children, also ambiguous. Examination of these constructs will focus on concepts of children as precious and sacred, as innocent, as deserving an individual emotional bond, as different and risky, and finally as worthwhile.

The study carers construct the foster children not only as precious but generally as morally more 'needy' than their own birth children. There are, however, individual foster carers who are exceptions. Grace, arguing that she is child-centred anyway, explains to a 12-year-old that she is not prepared to change her way of life, 'So *you* will have to fit in . . . I'm just a very as-you-see-me-is-what-you-gets'. But minority statements and sentiments like this have to be searched out.

As previously noted fostering produces significant changes in lifestyles, routines and habits as carers adapt to life-looking-after-other-people's-children. Meg, now relegating housework and gardening to second place in favour of children's needs, recounts how new foster carers:

> were asking things about these kids adjusting to a different – I said, 'it's not the *kids*. We're the ones that got to adjust' . . . we're the ones got to do the adjusting and changing, and we have to do it for every different child we get.

Meg's construction of each adolescent is that they are individually so precious that she must make personal adaptations to suit their uniqueness. In other transcripts this is apparent in small but significant ways. Cyril allows the foster child to choose the television programmes, even if Cyril himself watches Teletubbies rather than sport. John simultaneously turns a blind eye to the untidiness and a deaf ear to the noise. Kathleen used to 'watch all the soaps' but no longer has time nor opportunity. Stuart now:

> stand[s] on railway stations . . . watching trains . . . I've changed. I've become interested, for him, in trains. I don't go to discos, *they* like going to discos, we go to discos. So there *is* a change there comes from somebody being sensitive to what their needs are . . . and it's a joy . . .

None of them want to go and play table tennis. I play table tennis. I haven't met one that wants. . . .

These five carers are all certain that, for them, fostering is about prioritising the needs of the foster child at the expense of both their own wishes and, as already noted, possibly those of their own children. Foster children are so precious, their needs so sacrosanct, that on occasions there appears to be no consideration of the carers' own rights or desires. The final vignette (see pp. 119–120), the removal of two foster children because of an allegation, makes clear that the allegation is false. Yet, whilst struggling with the dilemma, not all the female carers automatically gave their husbands precedence. Mary, who is devoted to her dogs, remembers when one closed its mouth around a child's arm. She spontaneously thought, 'That's it. My dogs have got to go'. The personal investment in the foster child is deeper; the foster child is worth any sacrifice. But in order to understand this it is necessary to further deconstruct the concept, commencing with foster children constructed as innocent.

For some foster families, children's exclusion from school, offending, drug experimentation, graffiti and damage to the home, verbal and physical abuse can on occasions become the material of everyday life. Whilst each of these are mentioned in interviews, very few describe children in ways that are critical or judgemental. The transcripts reveal few negative accounts. Grace, as a minority example, mentions that children 'could be devious' (in relation to the false allegation vignette). The study carers' constructions of both the children that they look after, and the hypothetical foster children in the vignettes, are usually as innocents and as lacking moral agency.

For some this construction is allied to problems with the local authority and an emphasis on children's rights. Ali Shah tells of different children threatening to complain to their social workers about his family:

We like to do as much as we can but when you see this behaviour in a child, that does hurt you. That's a bad experience I would say and they *all* do it. *Not* one child. And it's not fault of a child it's the fault of social services . . .

[and upon consideration of resignation as a foster carer]

I say, what's the fault of the children? You know, we might be able to help somebody who really needs a good home. So why deprive him or her because of the system?

Ali Shah's experience is that if foster children's demands/'rights' are thwarted they complain to the department. His explanation is that this behaviour is overencouraged by social workers and he therefore exonerates the children from blame. On occasions he and his wife have found the attitude of the department so inexplicable that they have considered resignation but continue to foster in the belief that the children are not culpable. His construction of the innocence of children rests on his laying blame upon the local authority.[1] Something of this is echoed by Steve. He and Georgina both work yet the ten-year-old foster boy they had for weekends is now placed full time:

> I mean we haven't got a problem with Dylan, but it's just the mechanics of it just aren't working for us . . . I don't really think he's a problem. He's, behaviourally he's got, you know, a few idiosyncrasies that school is obviously trying to sort out . . . it's not Dylan's fault that he's in that situation.

Like Ali Shah, Steve maintains that the problems of caring for a foster child stem not from the child, but from his past life compounded by the 'mechanics' of the local authority. Dylan is an innocent in the bureaucratic machinery; he cannot be blamed because they have been let down. Finding the department liable, both men therefore make a comparative construction of foster children as innocent and without moral agency. Likewise Sam lists years of problems, 'with the social services. That and the baggage that comes with the children, for example the parents. There are no problems with the children. Just huge problems with everything else'. Dealing with the department and the children's parents is problematic but he finds caring for the children straightforward. Nevertheless Laura's description of one of their foster children appears far from uncomplicated: 'He feels the world's let him down at the moment, everybody's let him down . . . he's smashed his bedroom up a few times but we still love him. And we don't *part* with him'.

For Laura there are reasons and explanations for all behaviours and these do not detract from her love of, or her commitment to, the foster child. Similarly Georgina speaks of not 'judging a child . . . it's not his fault'. Kelly remembers Nathan's disruption of school classes and her regular visits to mediate and encourage staff to treat with compassion rather than sanctions. She was certain that he required not more discipline but more understanding. Likewise Olivia notes that children in care, 'don't show any more different traits than normal children, except they're far more extreme and now, because you know what they're coming from, you cope with a lot more because you know their problems aren't their making'.

Olivia's fostering experience has taught her that all children have the same basic characteristics but environmental factors affect their dispositions and their behaviours. It is this conviction that leads to her construction of foster children as innocent. The wanton damage caused by Celia's foster child leads her to conclude that he was upset by his mother. All children have agency but, for these foster carers, this is distinct from moral accountability. Celia and Olivia, like many others, believe that foster children's unacceptable behaviour has an explanation. It is this 'explanation' that apparently maintains for many carers their construction of the child as innocent; as passive victims that have things 'done' to them. Most carers connect innocence/lack of moral agency with the child's life experiences. Janet, describing how eight-year-old Craig's behaviour reduced her to tears, explains that before he was placed with her, 'he sort of like moved from place to place bless him, so . . . you can understand why he's like he is'. Cyril, considering Craig's tantrums sums up, 'I mean you can't blame him, 'cos he's a foster child'.

This is clarified by Gordon reflecting on a child's dangerously violent outbursts:

> [W]e didn't know the *reason* why he was doing it, but we could understand it. There's a problem because he's away from his mum, or what happened to his mum, or whatever. So it's something in his past that's caused him to be like that. So that's not really his fault, so you can understand all that, so it makes it a lot easier.

These carers perceive each foster child as the sum of their life experiences, some of which are seen to have been highly disturbing. Thus, however unreasonable the child's behaviour it is because of these experiences and the child should be understood by them. The child cannot be held to account. This explanation holds currency for many situations. Margaret, missing Jamie who had held the family at knife-point, muses:

> It's a shame how he went because he didn't have a very good life really. Upbringing. I think that was a lot to do with it. It kind of twists them up in their mind . . . He's had such a lot to go through really with one thing and another. You can't blame the child. No you can't blame a child.

Lenin, cataloguing Karl's antisocial behaviour whilst they walked around town, (stopped an escalator, racist comments, broke display goods and caused offence in a café) concludes, 'As I say it's his age, it's his upbringing . . . but it's certainly his own circumstances as regards the learning disability and things like that'.

These extracts demonstrate that for all these carers the foster child is innocent, a victim of personal circumstances that are beyond the child's control. It is the adults in the child's life, birth parents, social care personnel, foster carers, who are accountable and morally responsible. Foster carers must work to understand the reasons for the child's actions, however antisocial.

This same belief is corroborated in some of the foster carers' comments on the vignette concerning the unfounded allegation from a foster child. Gordon posits, 'I think it's anything kids say. I know it's not really their fault, so you've got to try and understand that . . . adults have to work it out themselves'. He suggests that the child is without blame/fault and that the onus is upon the adults to interpret the underlying reasons for the child's statements. Margaret's response, having experienced an allegation herself, is:

Well it's just one of her little tales then. 'Cos they do, don't they? Children do. It's probably something like she wanted something and she couldn't get it and she made a little tale up. Yeah, they should have them back. Yeah. Yeah I'd have them back, yeah.

This resonates with Mo's 'I wouldn't reject them for one mistake they've done, they're only kids. Yeah, they're only kids'. Whilst Mary, having met two carers who had been suspended from fostering for 18 months because of allegations, explains, 'the boy had just, you know, got upset and, as kids do. You know kids'. Mary is certain that this notion of the innocence of children is understood and accepted. It is part of the everyday world of childhood.

Jackie postulates an explanation in relation to teenagers who, at a transitional time on the edge of adulthood, are being prepared for independence. Speaking of other carers on her scheme, she recounts 'horror stories' of young people not being treated as part of foster families but locked out all day and concludes, 'People have got to realise, you can't *do* that with these youngsters. Because they get into trouble if you do that'. Jackie's construction of the foster child as innocent depends upon their treatment by others, in this case other foster carers. She is removing agency from the foster children; their unacceptable actions are their response to adverse circumstances. It is therefore not surprising that, when relating problematic histories of her own fostered teenagers, she reflects, 'You feel, well where did I go *wrong*?' Foster children are not held accountable for their own actions. They are not responsible. Like many other carers Jackie apparently takes upon herself the blame for foster children's undesirable behaviour. This construction, in common with other carers, of the innocence of children, with whom they have no blood ties and over whom they have no legal rights, indicates committed, personal ties.

As noted, caring and parenting overlap at many points where foster children are concerned. Parenting is primarily a personal activity arising from the individual, idiosyncratic relationships between those involved. But foster children are bureaucratised children for whom there are rules and cautions (for example, the physical demonstration of affection) which may be in conflict with the foster carer's choices regarding parental agency.

There is scant evidence of foster carers constructing foster children as embryonic adults (see Richard, discussed below). Jackie, Lenin and Meg, who prepare youngsters for independence, construct them as dependent and needy, requiring understanding and love. The transcripts overflow with the vocabulary of emotionality. Keith reflects on his upset at leaving a child with another carer for 24 hours and the emotional exhaustion of wanting both to give the best to foster children yet, as instructed by the social worker, to remain detached:[2]

You can't say 'oh I'm going to be unloving, I'm going to be not unkind, I'm just come in the house that's it, go to bed', you know, you can't do it . . . you've got to have feelings. I mean I think you've really got to . . .

[And on the foster child's initial rejection of him] It was quite upsetting, he brought me to tears once . . . I was really upset. I thought, what am I doing wrong?

Keith's tie with the young child is readily apparent. Its expressive component means that he is unable to behave in a pragmatic way, leave Timmy with another carer, act in a kind but indifferent way towards him and believe that rejection is general rather than personal. Foster children are constructed as deserving love.

Equally Emma contemplates preparing herself for the foster child's departure and knows that 'it will be hard and I'll probably sob'. Ruth describes how she arms herself with popcorn, ice-cream and the television's 'weepy film and pretend I'm crying because I'm watching the film' when children leave. Like Keith, Emma and Ruth construct themselves as foster-carers-who-demonstrate-caring in terms of their feelings of loss with each individual child.

Many of the accounts serve to demonstrate the positives of 'caring about' as foster carers construct themselves as moral caring beings. Louise criticises the social worker who observes, 'one thing you are going to have to do is sever this bond you've got with this child', when she believes that it is this demonstration of her 'caring about' that is beneficial to Victoria's well being. Similarly Mandy is clear that Timmy 'deserves to be loved' whilst Gordon is adamant that 'I think you've gotta just love unconditionally. I mean you've got to have that in your heart, you've just gotta'. This tenet of a particularistic tie and affection for each individual child is a common theme. Foster carers, looking after the children of others, know about exclusive loving relationships with specific children. Whilst it is said that social workers in the public domain give advice to 'sever this bond' and maintain a distance, foster carers in the private domain view themselves as intimately and emotionally close to each child. This is frequently demonstrated by the study carers' discussion of the vignettes. Margaret's reaction to pressure to accept an additional child is acceptance, 'otherwise it seems a shame they could lose her'; rather than consider the dilemma as a principle, she responds to the personal needs of a particular child.

Several of the carers disclose personal, emotional relationships with children they care for and about.

[I]t tears you emotionally a lot [of] times simply because you may have a child that you become particularly attached to or that you think needs certain therapy or care and you can't get it. And *that* causes quite a lot of emotions . . . *with yourself*.

(Brian)

I do get emotionally involved with them. I cry for them, I'm happy for them, whatever . . . and it *is emotional*. You want the best for them . . . You've *got* to get emotional, if you don't get emotional that means you're cold and if you're very cold then the kids are going to pick up on this.

(Jackie)

Looking after other peoples' children demands, and gets, an emotional response from these carers. Their construction of this may vary; the emotion may be linked to personal attachment, wanting to obtain particular services for an individual child, striving for a child's success or a means of helping the young person in a specific way. But the net result is often experienced as a cost to the carer in their representation of foster-carer-as-emotionally-caring in response to their perceived need of the child for a particularistic tie.

Meg considers her relationship with Wes, a young offender, explaining, 'I loved that boy, still do', and continues with her married son Rick's views of her fostering career:

I think Rick was jealous because I think he knew, because I had a lot of feeling for Wes. You know, I really did. I mean I've broken my heart over Wes. I've sat and cried my eyes out. And I've taken him back no end of times.

For Meg the costs are not only her own emotional pain over Wes but also the hurt to her only child. Implicit within her transcript is that each foster child needs a mother's love which she should provide. Nonetheless, not all of the boys she fosters receive such a close relationship. One boy reported her to social services for calling him names to which she comments, 'Wes would never, have ever, really reported me. I think, I mean, I could hit Wes. Wes wouldn't, he would just accept that as part and parcel'. Meg's care of Wes is 'an expression of moral commitment that requires people to behave towards one another in caring ways' (Brannen *et al.*, 2000: 4); it would be uncaring if he reported her. Furthermore she constructs a true emotional bond as overcoming all obstacles and breaching boundaries including both foster care rules and the rights of looked after children.

Jackie's experience with a boy who was out until three o'clock at night demonstrates her particular construction of the strength of emotional ties with fostered youngsters.

When I started telling him off he said to me, 'What do you care?' he says, 'you're only my carer'. With that I just shoved him against the wall and said, 'I bloody *do* care else I wouldn't be in this state'.

Unexpected, (un)controlled emotion regarding foster children is also highlighted in Kelly's interview:

I think the job of fostering is so emotionally draining . . . in each of our children it has raised such strong emotions . . . You're not prepared for that. You're prepared for their difficult behaviour but not how to handle being torn and having strong feelings. Actually you get feelings that you've never felt before, like I've felt. I've actually felt like hitting and I've never felt like that before over anybody. But Roy brought that out which is frightening. Everything becomes more extreme.

Emotionality is linked with irrationality. Keith wants to return from work every day and 'not be unkind', nor so emotionally involved that he will shed tears. Kelly frightens herself with the strength of the feelings of caring whilst Jackie reports herself to the social services because she has physically pushed a teenager. All of these extracts confirm the connectedness of the carers with the foster children.

Some of them demonstrate this in intimate practical ways. Celia remembers a baby 'like our very own' who sat on her husband's knee to eat from his plate, whilst Hope recalls the imperceptible growth of her love for Lindsey:

I might give her something to eat and she doesn't want it, 'oh well I'll finish that bit off'. That's what I'd do with Arash and Zeeba [birth children]. So it's those sort of things . . . there's no *pause* now whereas before we would pause about certain things, and so the boundaries would be the same I think now as I had with my own children.

Both are explaining the experience and the complexity of the connectedness between themselves and the children in terms of the dayliness of life. For them it is the detail of their care that expresses the emotional content. Much of this parallels our ideas about mothering and caring in what is referred to in short-hand terms as family life. Foster children are constructed as deserving love in similar terms to carers' own children. It is a construct that includes a full range of emotions. But the transcripts reveal that carers also construct foster children as 'different' and as 'risky'.

Whilst stipulating that all children deserve parity and are the 'same', 'a child is a child' (Cyril), carers also admit that foster children are 'different'. Mandy, Georgina and Stuart all point to the discrepancies from having no shared past. Jackie encapsulates these dilemmas as 'You wouldn't have rules for your *own* children, you have *understandings*', and enumerates:

[L]iving in a foster family is different because you have to treat the kids certainly in lots of different ways. The things you can't do . . . this *boundaries* and obviously I mean, like a lot of carers, I probably cross from time to time, you know. You *know* you leave yourself open to things.

Jackie understands that she leaves herself open when she pushes a foster lad and simultaneously pushes the boundaries. But for some carers having to concede the differences and act upon them causes problems. Stuart and Hanneke's family comprises children from her first marriage, plus their own son and the foster children, so 'fairness' is important. Stuart believes that different children require bespoke handling and objects to the fact that they have few sanctions where foster children are concerned. Hanneke explains that if foster children are with them for a short time then the family can cope with difference, but for stays of several months there has to be parity. Khanm Shah makes explicit how foster carers are obliged to treat the children with difference, 'Own children, you're free to tell them anything but foster children you have to watch not to shout them and not to touch them'.

Several carers comment that, for a bureaucratised child, differences are of necessity built in. Ruth describes them as 'legally set apart' and identifies that taxiing them to school overtly confirms difference. Isambard observes that the social services' scale of pocket money (regarded by many as over-generous) serves to preserve differentials. Dick, remembering how foster children were stigmatised when his parents fostered, considers that the view of the general public remains unchanged as people comment, 'cor you must be a marvellous person taking on a job with some child like that', or 'you're gonna have nothing but problems'. This public construction of foster children as difficult is experienced by Georgina, thwarted in her efforts to organise day-care. Her daughters' childminder refuses explaining that her husband fears Dylan might break the computer: 'foster children have this stigma'.

Generally the carers struggle to make sense of whether they construct foster children as the same as or different from their birth children. Whilst Ann is probably at one extreme overtly acknowledging differences, Grace represents the other, ostensibly denying disparity – although, as the following extract demonstrates, she does understand that foster children are different. She recounts how three siblings said:

> 'Don't tell anybody that we're your foster children. You must tell them we are your cousins . . . if when we were asked we'll say that we are your cousins and you are my Nanny Grace'. And that's what they said. Nobody told them to do it . . . So I mean, they have the sense to consider difference and all that.

Most of the carers strive to make sense of the positioning of the foster children within their families. Hope's response to the vignette concerning the foster child who bullies the carers' birth child is that to prevent retaliation by the victim is to build in discrepancy. Ali Shah's experience is that it is the social services department that insists upon differential care. He maintains that he treats foster children as his own but is criticised for the equivalence of his care, for example permitting small children in the marital bed. Many carers mention the social services' instructions and prohibitions regarding close physical contact with the children and the need to use what are referred to as 'Safer Caring' practices. Some of them regard aspects of fostering as potentially risky and construct the children as possibly threatening to their fostering status. Foster children are seen to present several risks. Foster carers know that they may be blamed if there is any physical harm to a child; there is the risk of becoming emotionally attached and there is also what the foster carers construct as the 'problem' of children's rights. Foster children are also constructed as different and dangerous because potentially they may make allegations against carers, criminally offend within the foster home or pose a threat to the stability of the foster family.

Brian recalls how Marcia's manipulative behaviour threatened his marriage, whilst Georgina currently struggles to decide where her loyalties lie when care of the foster child conflicts with family needs:

> My mother, who has done the fostering, and my friends said, 'you work full time, why are you thinking of getting this extra burden on?' And I said, 'because . . . I was assured that it wouldn't affect my work and it would be possible to do both' . . . We never go anywhere anymore unless we take Dylan and I, talking to a best friend and she said, 'All you do is think about Dylan. You don't think about Steve [husband] and how he's feeling and you're sort of saying well, we've started this so we finish it. But . . . if it's affecting how you listen to him'. So I've had to make a big decision *and the family I've got*, if you like, are the important ones and there's no good if I'm going battling along on my own with no assistance from anybody else.

Georgina had hoped to assimilate a foster child within her current family comprising her two daughters and a new husband. But, as explained elsewhere in her interview, the family are tightening their boundary and excluding Dylan. Although Georgina constructs Dylan as a victim of circumstances, nonetheless his presence in the family has generated a threat. She has given him priority above her husband and daughters. She is forced to reflect upon this and to choose between the past equilibrium of her family unit or its destabilisation through fostering.

Other carers demonstrate resistance if there is a threat to their families. Celia refuses parental contact for Micah in her home, fearing a risk to her birth children. She and Laura have requested removal of boys who aggravated their own daughters and were 'breaking up the family' (Celia). Although foster children may be frequently constructed as so precious that their needs come before those of other family members, nevertheless there are occasions when, if the foster child poses a threat to the stability of the family, the sacralised child may be sacrificed. But the reasoning behind such decisions is based upon the construction of the foster children as exemplified by Jackie and Richard:

> Jake was alright but as I say he stole and I don't, I just can't accept that. Well I can accept it from the likes of the three downstairs [young foster children] . . . [because of] the age group really. Someone who's sort of like 7 or 8 they take it . . . as long as they realise what they're doing. When you get to about 10 to 12 then you know it's wrong, but you know it's one of those things, you either accept it or you don't. But from a 16 plus, and Jake was going on 18 and that is, to me, is totally unacceptable . . . so he left. It was only a matter of pence but it's, it was the principle.

Here, Richard's moral construction of foster children is age-defined. Children aged '16 plus' are constructed as ethically accountable adults, so Jake's behaviour is seen as a threat to Richard's principles, whilst the younger foster children (in contrast) are confirmed and constructed as without moral agency, as 'natural innocents' (Ribbens, 1994). Jackie's reaction to theft, and the consequent eviction, is more ambivalent:

> She stole my cheque book . . . before you ask, yes I *do* still see her and yes I do still talk to her. Any *major* money I must admit I do keep locked up in my bedroom and I've got like a filing cabinet.

Jackie's construction of this adolescent is that it is the behaviour, rather than the person, which is unacceptable. Nonetheless fostered young people are sufficiently risky to warrant locked filing cabinets and the safekeeping of cash. But for nearly all the foster carers it is not the safekeeping of their goods that causes them to construct the children as risky but the safe-guarding of their reputations and their public integrity. They are very aware of the risk of complaints from the children against them, as Hanneke demonstrates:

> [A]ll these kids want fantastic, you know, *named* [designer] things and they just demand so much that the demand outstrips the, both the finan-cial and the physical . . . I mean they almost threaten you, and you know, 'You're neglecting me. You're not – ', like the child that we had, she said . . . I don't buy her any trainers. It's not that I didn't *buy* her any trainers. I just didn't buy new Nike trainers. But it comes *back* to the social worker . . . So, I mean then you have, 'So-and-so said she needs some trainers and she hasn't got any'. I said, 'No that's not the truth at all. I told her that she can have some trainers but she just can't have any Nike trainers'. Oh, you know. But it has to be checked out every single time and I think, 'Oh this is so tiring'.

Elsewhere in interview Hanneke notes how physically and emotionally exhausting fostering can be. Here she details how the 'demand outstrips the, both the financial and the physical' supply and that 'we are left continuously checked up on, having to explain ourselves'. Hanneke's experience is that fostered children's unmet demands can become complaints which social workers must investigate. She constructs foster children as risky because allegations about her care count against her reputation as a moral person.

Meg's attitude towards allegations or complaints about her care is forthright. The current teenager has resisted her offers of nurture; in anger she 'just turned round and told him that I'd never known such a whingeing, whining boy. I couldn't help it'. He read out to his social worker a written statement detailing her name-calling:

> They were no more than what I would have said to my son, or anybody else, the way he was carrying on. But he had written everything down, word for word and I would *not* have him back in the house again. I won't because *of* that.

Meg steadfastly states that her construction of foster children is that they all require 'love': her offer of a personal particularistic tie. She regards them in the same way as her own son; they receive parity of treatment with regard to both love and discipline. It is therefore unacceptable if the fostered child reports her in a way that she constructs as both unfeeling and distant, in a bureaucratised manner. This is not the relationship that she offers and he is therefore risky. In interview she is adamant about the importance of fostering to her way of life so youngsters who behave in this way are constructed as a danger to her well being. Studies of stepfamilies reveal an ethical imperative that constructs the child as without moral agency and the adult as fully morally accountable.[3] But, for the minority of study carers, this is not non-negotiable. So Meg, who changes her routine for each fostered adolescent in the belief that she must attest the love that they all need, when threatened, can demonstrate an ethic of self-care.

Several study carers had experienced investigations into allegations regarding their care. They were aware that behaviour perceived as inappropriate by the foster children might result in their removal from fostering. Training instructs that everyday events like bath time and bedtime are potentially risky situations. Social workers deconstruct foster children from children-needing-care-and-families and reconstruct them as children-who-could-be-dangerous to foster carer careers. Most of the participants in this study admit this redefinition, even if they also resist it. Many criticise the impracticalities; they cannot both take one child in the car to school or both be available at bath time, and argue the negative effects upon children and childhood. Brian protests that he always played with the children but can only do so now when Tricia is present and complains that, 'It's spoilt childhood'.

Changes in behaviour are overt. Steve states, 'we're really conscious of the nudity thing' and Simon wears a dressing gown if he wants a drink at night, even though no one is around. Ann, who describes her two foster boys (aged eight and ten years) as 'pseudo adopted', tells how:

> We both kiss them goodnight in the bedroom but we do it with the door open. And we don't sort of take *ages* over it. I wouldn't *sit* and watch television on my own in their bedroom on their bed. But then we sit and watch television in the living room, the four of us, and give them a cuddle then and everyone else can see what we are doing.

Harold clarifies:

> Last Sunday morning at half-past six my granddaughter was staying, jumped in our bed because she does and in comes Ruby the foster child *who jumps* on the bed and follows her and Kathleen [wife] gives me a nudge and I have to get up so that I'm not in bed in any way at all with these two, with the little girl, because in the book it says I *mustn't be in bed*, so I had to get straight up, get dressing gown on. I have to get up at half-past six on a Sunday morning!

As these extracts show, foster children are constructed as so risky that foster carers have to both watch their behaviour and be seen to be transparent in following 'the book'. The internalised public gaze is, for foster carers, overt monitoring, though Simon, echoing many carers, protests that social services do not support these behavioural changes by giving carers essential information about the children:[4]

> [B]efore they come to us, saying about their backgrounds and what they *have* done and what they *haven't* done, taking drugs etcetera . . . we never knew they had a drinking problem, you don't know if you've got one with sticky fingers . . . that sort of thing. It won't change us but we'll know what we'll be looking out for.

He constructs children as risky, and even though his household has been investigated for serious allegations he nevertheless constructs this risk as manageable, something they can 'look out for'.

Not everything is manageable. Carers with long-term placements are offering children a 'family' for life. As the carers get older, will their blood children accept responsibility? Mo is conscious of this for Lindsey, a foster child with profound disabilities:

[W]e have taken this responsibility, it's a huge responsibility for the future . . . the condition she's in, is she getting worse or better? But . . . even if she stays the same? . . . I'm getting older . . . and less energy, less patience. Hope's going to be the same and Lindsey's getting bigger and needs more attention, or more looking after. Obviously yes it does make me *think* . . . it is something yes that *worries* me . . . Zeeba [birth daughter] asked me once, 'Oh Daddy when you are old or even dead who's going to look after Lindsey?' and I said, 'I really don't know yet'.

Lindsey is a foster child but Mo does not consider her a public responsibility. She is a personal anxiety because he cannot plan for uncertainty; there is no resolution. Whilst this is also true for birth parents, Mo and Hope have voluntarily renounced 'normal' expectations of leaving dependency behind. For him commitment to a foster child provokes unease. Like most of the carers, Mo, in his own way, constructs his foster child as different and as risky. Yet only one (known) couple were considering resigning from fostering. Somehow all the carers, alongside the 'risk', construct the foster children as rewarding.

Kelly reminisces about a holiday with their foster child and his friend:

That was so lovely. It was more rewarding taking Shaun with us . . . you just got so much back from him . . . I remember taking him to the dolphin show . . . We didn't watch the dolphins . . . we watched Shaun . . . their little faces were alive and Shaun's, his mouth was wide open and his eyes were like this [demonstrates]. We just sat and watched *them* . . . and that for us meant so much . . . Shaun who came with hardly any clothes. I was having to wash his clothes daily . . . but it was lovely. That was *so* rewarding to do that. That for me means a lot. That's the sort of thing that makes it all worthwhile.

For Kelly and Clive the enchantment of childhood means that whatever they give the foster children is more than reciprocated. Ribbens McCarthy and colleagues (2000) review work on negotiated care responsibilities and definitions of childhood and argue that the care of children is independent of reciprocity. Yet for Kelly the daily washing of Shaun's clothing is constructed not only as a labour of love but a gratifying task. Elsewhere her transcript details the emotional pain of fostering but she constructs the foster children in such a way that this extract shows that meaningful times are reparative, 'makes it all worthwhile'.

This construction resonates throughout other interviews. Keith, who normally celebrates his birthday at a restaurant describes how, instead, they took Timmy, age four, to a family pub: 'it made up for it because we enjoyed watching him, you know, we get enjoyment out of seeing him mixing . . . but I think you get enjoyment every day'. Timmy is not constructed as spoiling the birthday meal, but as a source of happiness. Brian echoes this:

[Y]ou get a lot of rewards from the children . . . been a delight over the years really to foster pre-adoption babies . . . you are actually giving somebody *something* and you feel personally that you, I think it makes you feel quite good sometimes, you're actually able to give a couple that have been longing for a baby and can't have one themselves such a lovely present. So in that sense I think you get your rewards.

For Brian the babies are personally donated gifts. He is sharing the enthralment of childhood when this act of giving not only affords him pleasure but makes him feel rewarded. Celia remarks, 'some of the children are really loving and, you know, you get your credit through them in a way'. Her interview also reveals life-as-foster-carer as difficult but, like Brian, there are compensations derived through her construction of the children as a source of credit. Janet constructs herself as the debtor in the transaction, 'what you give up would never outweigh what you actually get in benefits'.

Likewise Mo is certain that the balance is in his favour. He explains that as Muslims his parents interpret fostering as 'buying a piece of heaven for myself you know, but really the *pleasure* Lindsey give us, yeah, it is more than, you know, what really heaven for us, if there is such a thing or not, I mean that's her smile'. His construction of their foster child, who requires 24-hour care, is not that she earns him his place in any afterlife but that her presence and her smile gives him heaven on earth. Because of Lindsey's profound disabilities this is likely to be an emotional 'heaven' because of her sentimental value.

Other carers construct the value of foster children in more practical terms. Daisy, with no birth children, depicts the daily routine of foster-child-care as 'exciting. I know it sounds silly', whilst Frances, awaiting her first adolescent, muses, 'they'd each bring their own personality and I, I hope that we'd be able to interact with them . . . so I think we would gain a great deal'. Although uncertain, Frances constructs the foster children as of value and as contributing to the household so that there is, for her, a net gain. The unknown children will give them new personalities to learn to understand; fostering offers personal growth through relationship as, 'neither of us want to retire. We don't want to sink into taking life too easily . . . I think we're ready for a challenge'.

Her particular construction of foster children is as new life for a retired couple; foster children supply a purpose. This same construction is evident elsewhere: Alfred, Jackie, Simon and Meg also describe foster children as providing personal tests. Tricia unpacks the construction:

[Y]ou find things within yourself that you are good at or you've been able to do that you never thought you would . . . for instance, to care for special needs children that I always . . . used to find quite hard in even going near to. Yes that's been quite a realisation for me. Quite difficult.

Foster children are constructed as worthwhile for Tricia because they enable her to do more, to overcome former obstacles, to prove particular things to herself. It is a symbiotic relationship where both parties benefit. Other carers speak of their personal achievements through the children. Yvonne sums up for several with, 'if you can put one child on the right road you've done something in your life', whilst Brian considers it a 'vocation . . . doing something worthwhile'. Two carers reflect upon the ways that fostering has produced self-change. Ruth has learnt to drive whereas Stuart had achieved an ambition by becoming a role model. These carers construct foster children as important because fostering provides the catalyst for reinvention. Daisy, a new carer, is clear that this is her raison d'être:

> I sort of wanna change my life, I *want* to do it, I want that fulfilment you know. I want to be able to cook dinners for children . . . I *wanted* to change . . . there was nothing I *didn't* want to change . . . There's nothing really I'd want to stay the same you know.

Fostering makes life worthwhile and gives it moral value. Children offer change, drama, events and enchantment. She will become a 'family' with opportunities for personal growth. Some of these constructions are replicated in the interviews with Khanm Shah, who found caring for the children of others educational, and with Alice who discovers that having a foster child:

> makes the brain work more as well because you tend to get mentally lazy because you don't have to think very hard because she [birth daughter] knows what she's doing, she knows her routine and you don't have to get involved with social workers and health visitors and group meetings and so, it sort of wakens the brain up and you have to start thinking about things a bit.

Whilst other studies suggest that parents are deskilled by experts and that the impact of educational, medical and welfare professions on (Australian) households leads to the disenchantment of the home (Richards, 2000), Alice finds continuous negotiations with professionals mentally stimulating. Foster children are for Alice, as for Daisy and Khanm Shah, constructed as worthwhile.

Both Hope and Tricia construct foster children as so worthwhile that they consider a super-efficient form of fostering, a quasi-professional fostering. Hope's ambition is to leave nursing in order to care for more foster children. Tricia feels that she already offers a highly proficient service negotiating daily with health and social services professionals for children with special needs. Three of these were terminally ill and Tricia struggles to make sense of her part in their short lives:

[I]t gives me, a sense of, I don't know that satisfaction is the right word, having been able to do that. To offer that. To see it through, complete it, if that's the best and the only way it could have been. It's really difficult to describe actually.

Tricia tries to explain how she derives a personal satisfaction from looking after children who die in her care. Like Ali Shah, Hanneke and Dick, she portrays herself as 'offering' something to the children of others; as expressed by Georgina, 'I wanted to do my bit, not just give to charity, actually do something'. For these carers foster children are constructed as practical ways of repayment. Janet and Hope construct foster children as victims of society in need of rescue, whilst Lenin says his foster child, 'is ever so clingy, you know, he doesn't want to go out without me sort of thing, which is nice for me'. Sometimes the symbiotic relationship, the reciprocal bargain, allows for every foster child's loss to be a foster carer's gain, 'it's nice'.

Many carers relate that they foster because they want children (if they have none) or more (if they already have a family). Hope, Miranda, Louise and Alice want to add to their families whilst Margaret gains extended kin: 'I call myself a grandmother, foster grandmother now. I regard this little one [aged 16 years] here as *my* grandson. I did Jamie and I did Shaun'. In this regard carers construct the foster children as blood relatives in order to maximise their idea of family; foster children may make the experience of 'family' more real. Hope and Mo hold family conferences with their birth children in order to explore 'how fostering is for them', whilst Mary (with no birth children) rejoices that her previously uncommunicative husband now daily discusses the foster children with her. She also experiences an unanticipated bonus at work as fostering,

> opened my life . . . When I was at work one day and people are talking about their kids and their grand-kids and I was completely out of it, I couldn't communicate . . . But I'm now part of a wider circle if you like, even though you know the children are only with me for a very short time, but . . . people come up to me and sort of say 'Have you tried this?' 'Have you gone?' and it's a whole different, you know, which I've never been involved in before you know and it's lovely.

Colleagues at work construct foster children as family and foster carers as real parents. Caring gives Mary a socially constructed identity.

The presence of the foster children has created changes which these carers construct as positive. Gordon describes his new foster-children-family as, 'I think all these things together make it kinda like a family, yeah, it could be a biblical definition of family'. As a born-again Christian Gordon is placing upon the foster children his highest accolade; he constructs them together with Emma and himself as a traditional, loving family. Emma notes that the presence of the foster children is causing Gordon to slow down in his business activities which she regards as positive.

Correspondingly some carers portray foster children bringing sought-after psychological change. Laura, whose mother committed suicide, constructs foster children as giving her life fundamental meaning: without them she would be '*Depressed*! . . . I thrive somehow. Stan [husband] always says "fill the house up with babies. She won't do the housework but she'd look after the babies"'. Meg describes herself as 'a bear with a sore head' between teenagers; Tricia recognises her 'need for being needed', and Celia explains, 'I enjoy helping them. I enjoy looking after them. And to me it's fulfilling a part of *my* life, having the babies. I don't want any more family for myself *but* I am getting what I need off these children'. For these carers the significance of foster children is constructed as giving life meaning. Mary, whilst recognising the physical and emotional exhaustion of fostering, concludes:

> [W]ith Damien [foster child] I was tense, but the other tensions, not like tension, yeah I suppose other tensions they've gone. It's, I am relaxed. I know that sounds a contradiction of terms, yeah it's done me a lot of good, I know it has. I've got a great deal out of it.

Thus whether it is to ward off depression, provide an aim in life, know that a need is being met, feeling fulfilled or contributing towards a more relaxed persona these carers all construct foster children as necessary for their own psychological well being.

Alongside these constructions, foster carers also give practical reasons for wanting to absorb other people's children into their families. Brian and Mike clarify that their wives are preoccupied with child care anyway. Some females may find that fostering offers a retreat from the working world; for Miranda, fostering solves her need to be at home for her own son:[5]

> I can support myself . . . and be at home for Ashley which is what I want to do . . . I can do that and also extend my family, 'cos I'd quite like to have more children, but I possibly can't afford it. You see I send Ashley to a private school and I have to be able to fund that so it probably means I can't afford to have another child.

Rearing children is now more difficult and demanding; parents feel obliged to provide the most advantageous conditions (Beck and Beck-Gernsheim, 1995), in this case private education. Miranda's decision to foster is therefore instrumental. Foster children are constructed as a double benefit for the household. Their presence provides the wanted child and the financial allowance contributes towards their cost.

Older carers construct as an additional benefit that the presence of the foster children is rejuvenating. Margaret is reminded of when her own son was a boy; Yvonne states that 'even at 68 I feel like 38' whilst Cyril exults that foster children 'make me feel 10 or 12 year younger'. Meg maintains that she knows:

> all the pop tunes . . . I *have* to, to keep up with it all . . . yeah it's kept me alive actually. It really has because I think that anyone can sit back and vegetate, can't they? I mean I'm 65 now and I really don't, I just don't *feel* 65.

Meg is talking of the value of youth and of the priority of childhood. Alongside this renewal several of the carers positively enjoy particular aspects of childhood. Gordon and Arthur take pleasure in 'having a laugh' whilst Harry, Kathleen, Mandy and Ruth relish playing with the children. As Ruth describes:

> I do get to play a lot. And I do like to play with small people and I like fun and games and I like going 'ape' on trips and things which *now*, as my two [birth children] are now adults I wouldn't have actually had. I would have had to go and live in this grown-up world.

Foster children are constructed as a reason, an excuse, for foster carers to go 'ape' on occasions so that they can (re)join children's worlds and remember their own uninhibited, creative, sensual personalities. These carers construct childhood as different from adulthood; it demands different ways of being which they access via foster children. Foster carers construct the children as meaningful; they construct benefits from their personal and intimate relationships with them.

Foster children provide a sense of family, not only for the carers' private lives but also for their public persona. These children demonstrate the power of enchantment as foster carers construct them as innocent, precious and sacred. But this construction of the fostered children is also crucial to the construction of their own moral value. Throughout the transcripts there is evidence that the foster carers construct themselves as moral people in contrast with the social services and as 'ideal' parents in contrast to the children's birth parents. Birth parents and the children's beginnings are constructed as flawed. This chapter has quoted Stan referring to the parents as 'the baggage that comes with the children', whilst Olivia excuses difficult behaviour 'because you know what they are coming from'. Both Celia and Margaret blame past experiences and Lenin explains Karl's antisocial behaviour with, 'it's his upbringing'. The birth parents of the fostered children are thereby constructed as immoral and the children's behaviour difficult but explicable.

Like Gelder's childminders, foster carers perceive 'love as the reward for work' (1998: 6). Gilligan (1995) views care as a relationship so that a care orientation changes the way people approach political and moral issues.

Life is made meaningful for the foster carers not only because the children are deserving of time, attention, love and understanding but because the carers' personal involvement with the child's progress via an intimate, individualised tie offers the carer opportunities for personal growth. The relationship flourishes best when it is symbiotic, or reciprocal, as some foster carers pursue an ethic of care of self in order to benefit the foster child. But fostered children are public children; they are bureaucratised children. As previously noted, Meg's teenager writes out his complaints against her for his social worker. This is in conflict with a family discourse of love and a particularistic tie, and so unrewarding that Meg emotionally rejects and physically evicts him. Bureaucratised children are therefore ambiguous. They are risky and different. This construction is shared by the children themselves, the social services, the general public and the carers. Nonetheless, the behaviour of foster children as bureaucratised children, if not condoned, is regularly constructed by their foster carers as 'explained' by their personal histories. Through different constructions with regard to the children, foster carers find rewards which confirm commitment. This is what makes foster children worthwhile and they in turn make life meaningful.

6 Conclusion

This concluding chapter reviews the research and its findings in order to note the connections between the substantive issues and their related theoretical perspectives. It then discusses these by way of broader sociological topics in order to contribute to current sociological debate about childhood, contemporary morality and individualisation. It concludes with some examination of its relevance for social policy.

The social work/social policy literature review indicates that, not only have the local authorities marginalised the foster care service, but foster carers have been undervalued. The search provides only a fragmented and incomplete picture with little original sourced material giving any priority to the voices of the carers. The dominant view is that of the local authorities, of social workers and policy makers. The reasons for this are complex but importantly include political choices and contractual control demanding large-scale research designs (Burgess, 1994). Pertinently, although there have been many research projects within the home there are particular inhibitions regarding this as notions of home include, not only a strong ethic of privacy, but a provision of identity to its occupier which confers power (Twigg, 1998).

Chapter 1 noted that it may serve organisational interests for the (less powerful) status of the foster carers to remain unchanged. Sometimes dominant ideologies which justify the status quo (the power of the social services) silence the voices of others (in this case the place of female carers within the private sphere) in order to define and validate a particular, potentially oppressive reality. Perhaps partly because of any or all of these factors, information from foster carers, usually focusing on the children, has been primarily sought through postal questionnaires. The first chapter therefore concludes that the voices of foster carers are usually peripheral to more powerful voices in foster care studies.

A review of the sociology literature considering concepts of public and private, care and the family, demonstrates that the lives of foster carers are precariously balanced at the margins of several conceptual worlds. The private sphere theoretical worlds of motherhood, childhood and the family are usually compatible but for foster carers the public world, via the local council, acts as a vital agent upon this nexus. It is this element which so significantly reshapes all three concepts in such complex and contradictory ways that it might be concluded that the management of this precariousness might prove (theoretically) impossible. Mapped onto these concepts, foster care emerges full of paradoxes, with the foster carers having ambiguous status and having to manage a lifestyle which, in theoretical terms, is full of conflict.

The purpose of this research is to examine how foster carers understand their world. As there are no obvious models for them this study analyses how different individuals make sense of fostering. The research is not concerned with discovering 'truths' about foster carers or evaluating what they do; it focuses on their diverse personal experiences and perspectives in order to appreciate how they make sense of their roles and their everyday lives. It explores the ways in which they comprehend their experiences of looking after other people's children by deconstructing their statements and searching for their meanings. Together with the carers, the research questions taken-for-granted assumptions about family life in order to hear/see how they understand and make sense of their social worlds. It looks at how foster-carer-selves are constructed and presented in particular ways at particular times.

The research shifts the focus from the cared-for onto the carers to analyse how foster carers construct the children that they look after. Children who are ambiguous because they are public and bureaucratised and whose needs the local authority demands should take priority. Foster carers want to care for children. Zelizer (1985) posits that wanted children are regarded as priceless and sacralised because they are invested with sentimental meaning. The local authority's expectation therefore fits with most foster carers' construction of the children as precious. Carers regularly adjust their personal lifestyles, and those of their families, to suit individual foster children. The foster child is frequently considered worth the sacrifice.

Unpacking the reasons for this construction reveals that foster carers do report unacceptable behaviour by children. Examples include violence, wanton damage, theft and deception. Nevertheless, this is generally detailed by the carers in non-judgemental, non-critical terms. This holds true for many of them even when children allege maltreatment by their carers to the social workers. Thus, frequently, threats posed by the foster children do not detract from their emotional value. Foster carers often blame social services for these allegations, linking them to the social workers' emphasis on children's rights. Children are bureaucratically constructed as active participants whose competence is underestimated by adults. But foster care has traditionally operated within a needs, not rights, framework. Foster carers must now accommodate both perspectives, although in general they continue to construct foster children as innocent and without agency. It is, for foster carers, an unquestioned, taken-for-granted assumption that foster children are passive victims and cannot be held to account. Generally carers believe that antisocial actions are the result of environmental factors; there is always a reason, an explanation and therefore an excuse for all behaviour.

This portrayal as non-accountable, innocent victims is regularly defined by reference to the children's pasts and to the negative actions, or inaction, of their birth parents. Foster carers, in positioning the child as innocent, thereby shape the foster child's parents as at fault and place themselves in contrast to birth parents. By this mechanism they construct themselves as morally superior; as ideal parents who, compared to the birth parents, put the child's needs first. Ribbens McCarthy and colleagues note the 'importance of contrasts as a narrative device that (has) the effect of implicitly constructing a moral identity for the teller' (2000: 9). In this study the foster carers' constructions of innocent children necessarily involves apportioning blame to both the social care departments and to the birth parents. Blame is rarely allocated to the foster children.

Many foster carers acknowledge guilt, and blame themselves when their foster children do not succeed; like mothers they believe that they are held to account for their children. Generally the study carers accept public and private responsibility for the children and talk of failure when there are disappointments. They expect to 'save' children via a particularistic tie; the intimate, personal relationship they have with each individual child. The foster carer sense of self is one of connectedness. Emotional boundaries overcome own-family boundaries as they take responsibility for the child, for their physical appearance, their general behaviour and their personal happiness.

Yet there are some foster carers who manage emotionality differently. They either discriminate between children, feeling a sense of pride for a selected few, or, because they are not the birth parents, do not take responsibility for the children's attitudes and behaviours. But they are a minority in this study. The majority position themselves as responsible for the children, with some risk as to whether they will enjoy the rewards or suffer great costs. They do not regard children as socially competent but accept accountability for both the children's current actions and also for their future happiness. Their lives are focused around their foster children even though they have no autonomy of care; each child brings with them a birth family and the bureaucracy of the social services. Foster carers must understand and account for all this complexity.

Foster carers believe that foster children deserve to be understood through love. It is unfair to withhold this even if they believe that social services expect them to maintain an emotional distance. Jamieson (1998) makes the point that feelings of love, and actions of love, are quite distinct; carers can demonstrate care/love in practical ways without always feeling love. But emotional involvement is described by the carers as essential for the child's well being even though, as they intimate, this may be detrimental to themselves. This exclusive bond with the child is considered by many carers to be so essential that, for some, it may jeopardise blood-family relationships within the foster care household. Connectedness may change emotional behaviours; it may lead to excluding treatment of the foster carer's own family and offer more inclusive treatment to the foster child. But changed overt behaviours are also required to manage risk; foster children are different and can be dangerous.

Foster children are bureaucratised children. Their lives are circumscribed by rules, regulations and rights. Foster carers keep daily diaries on foster children's activities, attend meetings and accept into the home officers of the local council to monitor the child and survey the family. All of this affects foster carer decisions about the child's status within the household. Whether the child's presence is constructed in terms of being an 'insider' and 'same as', or 'outsider' and 'different from' the foster carers' birth children, these concepts and the carers' explanations for their decisions are multilayered and complex. Automatic construction of the foster child as 'insider/the same as' is cautioned by a subtle combination of the carer's belief that the fostered child deserves more in a bid to make up for past damaging experiences, reinforced by the reality of bureaucratised children's rights. The carer's construct these as giving the children power and thereby making them 'different from' and 'outsiders'. Foster carers must continually reposition themselves to cope with these paradoxes and ambiguities.

Nonetheless, most carers continue to foster (Sinclair *et al.*, 2004; Triseliotis *et al.*, 2000) whatever the general difficulties or personal problems of their situation, because of and for the sake of the children. Implicit in the transcripts is that looking after other people's children gives a real sense of family for those who have no children, or whose children have left home or who cannot afford more birth children. These extra children promise the total enchantment of childhood. Carers are certain that the children enrich their lives with happiness, rewards and credits, and 'heaven on earth'. For many, the children also offer opportunities for the carers' personal growth. Foster care is constructed, by different carers, as educative and providing challenges with the prospect of realising a sense of achievement. This contrasts with some research of caring for children which finds that, on occasions, it is stories of despair and difficulty which people may be most eager to tell (Gillies *et al.*, 2001). All the study carers construct fostering as worthwhile, whatever its tensions and difficulties.

Tensions and difficulties within the foster family household are primarily the result of the public world intrusion into and onto what is understood as the private lives of foster families. Bureaucracy's primary concern is the families' fostering status, and carers find that their own 'private/personal' non-fostering lives are eclipsed. The activity of fostering cannot be easily contained; it spills into the rest of life. Paid work lives may prove incompatible as fostering demands flexibility and adaptability. Time is affected; families become tied into the foster child's timetable of continuous demands. Foster family life may become dominated by current time as the unpredictability of events in the foster child's life prevents planning. Becoming a foster carer can involve spatial change (house extensions, modifications) and social change (no alcohol, child-centred activities). It affects relationships as confidentiality rules regarding the children inhibit openness between friends and relatives. Many foster carers construct their social lives mainly in relation to other carers who are empathetic to the often unsympathetic behaviour of unruly fostered children. Thus foster carers find that they redraw personal friendship boundaries. Fostering becomes for most a new caring identity.

'Carer' is a professional label, a public label, and does not denote family membership as does 'parent'. Foster carers must balance these two identities in relation to each fostered child. The care identity is implicit in both roles; being a foster carer is an uncertain category, more than carer but less than parent. The subjective experience of foster carers is as parents; they act as parents but have an ambiguous position. This unsure status is compounded by lack of both authority and control; foster carers rarely know how long a child will remain, or with whom the child maintains their primary allegiance: it may not be within the foster family.

Frequently foster families include both birth children and fostered children; dilemmas of equity and fairness are daily faced by these carers. Most carers say that they love the foster children as they love their own but know that they have to treat them with difference, if not deference, because of bureaucratic surveillance and the risk of allegations concerning their care. Most strive to manage this situation in a way which offers parity, but external pressures, primarily from the local authority, results in dissimilarity. When change is required it is frequently the birth children who have to adapt and possibly experience detrimental alterations in the quality of parenting; bureaucracy provides rules and regulations, but not practical solutions for children's care. Public, formalised bureaucratic structures do not sit comfortably with informal, loving, private households.

Bureaucracy's need for standard techniques means that care becomes a component of the regulatory system; it is converted from a human service into a commodity. Foster carers have to work with this rationale. Schofield and colleagues (2000) note the two, sometimes divergent, discourses of family and of bureaucracy that shape foster care. Studies of small care homes for the elderly (not so dissimilar from foster families) identify the gradual changes: from domesticity to institutionalisation, from normalisation to specialisation, from informality to regulation, from risk to security, from personal to professional and from privacy to surveillance (Peace and Holland, 1998). The social care department's bureaucracy can channel living to a point where foster carers perceive their household lives to be virtually owned by the local council. As they become increasingly 'professionalised' and 'institutionalised', foster carers must continuously account for everything. The foster home may no longer be 'a (private) haven' since it must be open to intrusion and inspection which can be experienced as hostile. Public bureaucracy and private family life are parts of different conceptual spheres with diverse values and principles. Bureaucratic efforts to regiment and regulate foster family lives can prove problematic.

There is, from the foster carers' perspective, a dominant theme of the (ab)use of bureaucratic power. Foster carers describe the social services as all powerful and themselves as powerless. They regularly position themselves discursively as without autonomy and construct their relationship with the department in terms of 'us' and 'them'. Edwards and colleagues, in examining reconstituted stepfamilies, identify that power in these families is not focused but diffuse (1999). Foster families are also reconstituted families and for them the power is spread across and between social services, the foster children's birth families and the foster family household. Legal discourse, via the Children Act 1989, gives the birth parents (rather than the foster carers) responsibilities and power so that, in law, 'there is no notion of "children need (social) parents"' (ibid., p. 758). This contributes to both the ambiguities of the child's place within the foster family and the complexities around the child's care.

Yet the normative standpoint of the foster carers is their intrinsic belief in increasing the foster child's stability via strengthening ties of belonging that will 'save' the child. It is this 'ownership' that is the foster carer focus for producing change and improvement in the lives of the children. In order to accomplish this the carers construct their own position as rescuers and as change-agents for needy children. They talk of provision for children via notions of 'family' and of 'home' in order to make a (positive) difference to them. They want to make them 'better' and to save them by incorporating the foster children into 'normal' (foster) family life. The majority of carers in this study construct, as the important component of their foster carer status, their personal influence to change and to save the fostered child. This is either via their own web of family-based loving relationships or an individual particularistic loving relationship with the child. Changing the child is centrally important to these carers. It gives their lives meaning and is thus personally gratifying. Fostering is not totally altruistic but reassures carers that they count.

The majority of study carers insist that money does not count.[1] For them family is not about rational economic exchange since (foster) children are beyond price and deserve unconditional love. Carers view themselves as giving their time for free and even those on fee-paying schemes continue to consider that caring is superior to money. A small minority are completely instrumental about the issue and want a wage-based foster care service. Many of the study carers consider themselves undervalued and exploited, but adamant that they wish to foster for the sake of the children.

In general, these foster carers confirm other findings (Sinclair *et al.*, 2000), describing the circumstances and the context of their fostering as fraught with complications. Although reporting that social care staff can be insensitive to foster families, there are no indications that any of the carers give up negotiating with the local authority in a bid to achieve preferential services for their foster child. Whatever the difficulties, frustrations and complexities of their situations only one study family possibly resigned from fostering through choice. The others establish their own coping mechanisms and find sufficient internal resources to confirm commitment. Although constructing their own situation as powerless, they create their own rewards through the children in relation to whom they position themselves as potentially very powerful in terms of the possibility of 'saving' them via an intimate relationship.

Lewis and colleagues' research review (1999) on individualism and intimate relationships between adults concludes that there have been few studies. This is also true concerning research on close relationships between adults and children. Giddens (2000) posits a (hypothetical) democratic family, where gender is a less salient issue between adults, and decision making includes negotiating with children. Thus equality, mutual respect and autonomy through communication should provide the family, and specifically the children, with stability. But for foster carers the issues concerning family and children are differently shaped. These are not the underlying concepts for their activities; this is not how they construct the foster child. Generally foster carers understand each foster child as needy, innocent and sacred and therefore deserving of protection (not consultation), which is provided via a particularistic tie and a notion of love. This discourse of protection seeks an empathetic response which provides the foster carer with a special relationship.

Beck and Beck-Gernsheim (1995) examine the importance of special relationships in a post-modern age; the need for intimacy and commitment in an increasingly unsure, shifting world. They hypothesise that, as the last half-century has witnessed new questionings of life with a constant search for individual meaning, there are no longer any certainties or explanations. Adults therefore need to find a sense of security and individual meaning through a particularistic relationship. There is a basic need for individuals to have a primary bond in order to develop a sense of identity. Relational aspects of family life are not on offer in the marketplace and individuals therefore seek this rewarding and satisfying relationship with another adult from elsewhere. But these 'pure relationships' (Giddens, 1992) are inherently fragile and cannot hold without mutual satisfaction: love is contingent rather than forever. Intimacy with another, in the context of commitment, promises fulfilment, but people must work at this the whole time, 'negotiating and deciding the everyday details of do-it-yourself relationships' (Beck-Gernsheim, 1998: 67). In this uncertain environment, relationships with (birth) children appear more secure and enduring.

There is no longer any material advantage to having a child but children have a 'psychological utility' (Beck-Gernsheim, 1995: 105); children can reward via intimate and holistic relationships. They therefore become very precious, a 'principle concern and a primary love object' (Jenks, 1996), as blood relationships offer some certainty and a fixed reference point. But for foster carers and foster children there is no blood relationship. Nonetheless there can grow an 'elective affinity' (Beck-Gernsheim, 1998: 66), a freely chosen act understood via the needs of the child which may, or may not, be reciprocated. If needed, each foster child becomes the all-important love object which makes life purposeful and provides happiness; they are regarded as priceless in terms of their meaningfulness and emotional value.

Yet relationships with fostered children are full of risk. Their tenure and primary alliances are always uncertain and their attitudes and behaviours can, at best, be unpredictable and, at worst, antisocial. Nonetheless carers appear to ignore the strong dichotomies presented by childhood, these 'extreme idealizations of child rearing juxtaposed with equally dismaying possibilities' (Walkover, 1992: 178). Conversely, analysis of the transcripts suggests that, for some carers, the more challenging the children's behaviours then the more they will protect and love.

Through love, foster carers construct themselves as individually necessary to each child. This raises a notion of self, an ethic of care of self, which is actually enhanced through the foster children. Current debates argue that an ethic of self-care, of individualism, is essentially selfish and in opposition to an ethic of child care thus suggesting that foster carers represent an anomaly in the modern world.

This requires consideration. The current decreasing birth rates in the West are of increasing concern (Boase, 2001; McRae, 1997). The reasons for this trend are several and complex; not least that paid work outside the home is regarded as fundamental to both self-esteem and the esteem of others. Today's post-modern, employed woman, in pursuit of individualism, described by Bumpass as the 'progressive legitimization of individual self-interest' (1990: 488), constructs children as undermining her sense of self. Invigorated by the culture of post-modernity (self-awareness and autonomy in private life), she is concerned with self-fulfilment, the valuing of risk and change and a morality centred around self-care which would be compromised by motherhood. Parenthood is therefore losing its ascribed status so the aspirations of foster carers for (more) children would appear to be in conflict with this particular trend.

Caring for foster children could be described as the ultimate challenge. Not only are they constructed as victims, needy and exhaustively demanding, but significantly they are bureaucratised, public children and their carers have circumscribed autonomy. There is also the disadvantage of different time orientations and competing time frames. Understandings of family include strong orientations to time past and to a future; children offer parents both futurity and nostalgia. Foster children bring no shared past and can promise no certain prospects of a future. Blood children not only ensure (re)presentation, but signify for adults hope and meaning in the future; they offer ongoing and infinite time. Foster children offer only finite time; foster carers must invest everything into their here and now. In a disenchanted modern world, the loss of the hierarchy which maintained the social disparity between parents and children now means that parents have to work at being loved (Jamieson, 1998), and Cunningham (1995) argues that child rearing is no longer about certainty but about negotiation. Even though relationships with children can be precarious, there is an expectation that foster children will give the lives of foster carers value. The meaning of life is loaded onto them via the relevance of a loving particularistic tie.

In this study, foster carers' moral selves are shaped by their construction of fostered children as vulnerable, innocent and deserving of care via a loving relationship that only they can provide. Walkover notes that 'parenting has been transformed from a duty to one's family, community, or country into an optional way of living' (1992: 183). Whereas the current trend is that many women do not want the responsibilities of parenthood and the duties of child care, foster carers positively seek these duties. Ribbens McCarthy and colleagues (2000) identify the significance of dependent children in upholding moral adequacy for (step) parents. Moral adequacy is not totally dependent upon children but once adults have young children there is a moral imperative that they not only take responsibility for any children in their care, but also accept that their needs are paramount.

The foster carers' pronounced ethic of care for others is prominent throughout many transcripts; they construct themselves as moral beings. Not only do they work to ensure that the children's needs are given priority but they do this in the face of problems and opposition from the social care department, other agencies such as schools, and the children's birth parents. Moreover, they give the children's needs precedence, regularly modifying their own lifestyles as required. It can only be that fostered children themselves represent something of significance. Foster carers must frame differently the dilemmas between the ethics of care of self and of caring for children.

For foster carers it can be argued that there is no potential collision of the two ethics (care of children and care for self), but a harmony as they complement each other. The ethic of care of self for the foster carer is tied in with the carer's self-esteem and self-identity. Looking after the children of others may be a service but more importantly, it is also a way of life whereby the foster carers describe their own interests as mutually compatible with caring. There is no collision or conflict. It is an essential part of what they are; it is a sense of self bound up with their love for the children and the motivation for their agency. In different ways they talk of the challenges provided by foster care; opportunities for education, for occupation, for mental stimulation and for emotional satisfaction. This describes a strong ethic of self-care but one that is not constructed in opposition to an ethic of child care. It does not become an immoral stance since it shores up and complements the ethic of care that serves children's needs. Foster carers construct fostering as providing a moral career.

Parenthood and family life is about being a moral person; Ribbens McCarthy and colleagues (2000) conclude that it is virtually impossible for a parent to relate an immoral tale with regard to children. As foster care is bound up with notions of being a moral person, can a foster carer express a negative view of the child as undeserving? Can they say that they don't like a child and experience them as unfulfilling? Brian and Tricia continue to grieve for the child whose behaviour threatened their marriage, and remain in contact with her. Celia, Laura, Grace and Stuart all describe requesting that children be placed elsewhere because of conflict with their birth children, but do not criticise the children concerned. Jackie maintains supportive contact with the young woman who stole her cheque book. Georgina intimates that she will have to request another family for their foster child because hers cannot provide the detail of care he requires; it is the fault of her family and not Dylan. But Richard evicted Jake 'on principle' and Meg insists upon the removal of a teenage boy. He has placed himself as a bureaucratised child by writing out a list of what she accepts as valid complaints against her care. This is set in a context where he rejects Meg's offers of kindness and daily grieves for his mother, refusing to allow Meg to replace her. As a public child with his own birth mother he repudiates his foster carer's overtures of nurturing and mothering. He has rejected the special relationship. It is thus perhaps only Richard and Meg in this study who consider that a child is undeserving of their care, and that it is therefore morally acceptable not to continue the responsibility. There are foster carers who will consider a foster child to be undeserving.

Beck and Beck-Gernsheim note that motherhood 'is felt to be a crucial and exceptional test of one's own character' (1995: 110) (although this may be a view from a particular class and ethnic perspective). Foster children are the definitive challenge, frequently requiring more understanding, patience, help and unconditional love than other children. Some foster carers put themselves through this test many times. Of the 27 foster households in this study, seven had fostered ten or more children, and three at least five. For them there have to be compelling reasons and motivations. It might be argued that as foster carers are not parents they do not consider themselves eligible for this 'character testing' except that the data demonstrates the converse. The majority feel personally culpable when they fail to access services required by their foster child or young people move on to, what the carers consider, unsatisfactory lifestyles.

Many foster carers accept accountability for the children. Their redefinition from (natural) foster parents to (professional) foster carers (within these accounts) means that they do not just measure the child's 'success' in public agenda terms of better health, education, achievements and behaviour. For foster carers the significance and strength of family discourse and family framework is such that they do not view the child as a bureaucratised, public, contractual child with defined rights. They embrace the child as needy; as a member of the family and as 'their' child. From this comes a notion of foster children that requires the carer to save them through love. Foster children represent the emotional value that makes carers feel not only responsible and important but also emotionally indispensable. Beck and Beck-Gernsheim (1995) posit that parents control their children under a cloak of love. This is confirmed by Gillies and colleagues (2001) who find that parental support may carry potential overtones of control and obligation. Certainly, for foster carers, loving the children provides a route to happiness and thus makes life meaningful. Giddens (1992) discusses the project of the self whereby individuals reflexively chart and rework their own life course and destiny. This requires an autonomous, discreet, rational being. Foster carers are possibly working with a different notion of self and a different project. Theirs is a relational self, based on interactive qualities continuously formed in connection with, and seeking emotional and physical empathy with, each individual fostered child.

Jamieson (1998), reviewing the literature on intimacy and parenting, considers whether motherhood necessarily involves a loss of sense of self. She quotes a US study of single mothers which concludes that women who intend to have a child avoid any supposed loss of individualism because it is motherhood by choice. This is certainly the position of foster carers who volunteer to look after the children of others. Foster carer is parenthood by choice. Foster carers look after children because the children of others confirm moral value.

A study by Barnardo's (1996) notes that children in the care system account for less than 1 per cent of their age group nationally but that they are massively overrepresented among those who become disadvantaged. Adults who have been in care are highly overrepresented in Britain's mental-health wards, unemployment figures and prisons (by 50 times), and 50 per cent of London's homeless adults have been in some form of public care. Only 9 per cent of looked after children in England get 5 GCSEs at grades A to C, compared to 54 per cent of all children, and fewer than 1 in 100 children leaving care go on to university.

Children in care are 10 times more likely to be excluded from school and 88 times more likely to become drug-abusers. Perpetuating the cycle, parents who have been in care are 66 times more likely to have their own children taken into care (Templeton, 2005). Buchanan and colleagues' (1993) examination of the data from the National Child Development Study suggests that children are disabled as much by the stigma of being 'in care' as the actual context of being looked after.

The complex, multilayered nature of this research data does not immediately offer straightforward policy recommendations for the foster care system. This qualitative research is concerned with exploring the views, attitudes and experiences of foster carers. Any dominant views and practices are not any more important than the others. The aim is to explore what gives rise to them all. It is arguably those findings which enable policy debate to progress.

Life-as-foster-carer in this study holds an unclear location, positioned on the edge of several (conceptual) boundaries; public and private worlds, neither volunteer nor colleague, not parent but more than carer. In life, those who have one foot in each camp are secure in neither; theirs is a precarious existence. Policy makers need to note the foster carer's situation, peripheral and excluded, lacking professional respect, marginalised from decision making and planning. Additionally foster carers are caught between two bureaucratic instructions which could be constructed as increasingly divergent. They are expected to meet the social services' objective of 'ensuring that all children are securely attached', whilst also recognising (where appropriate) the claims of birth families (DoH/SCG, 2000). For many foster carers, their work only makes sense if they truly love the children. Their accounts may challenge the discourse of social services. The ambiguity of their situation risks positioning them where they are alienated.

This research confirms major surveys that foster carers understand themselves to be alienated by social care departments; it demonstrates the ways that foster carers perceive themselves as 'othered' by bureaucracy. It may be that this contributes to their desire for intimate emotional attachments with the children and to their concentration upon the present. This can be in conflict with current established child-care practice which is to appreciate the holistic child including his/her valuable past. This study suggests a risk that some carers are taking foster children away from their personal/blood contexts. Foster carers have a significant role with regard to the developmental needs of children but perhaps some are seeking to do so on their own terms, ignoring the fact that many children have a past and a future independent of their carers. Best care for fostered children is normally considered to incorporate arrangements for them to see their birth families. Research, including this study, has shown that this is frequently an ambiguous, if not difficult, experience for foster carers (Schofield *et al.*, 2000; Waterhouse, 1992). This study demonstrates that fostered children provide meaning for the lives of some foster carers; this therefore has powerful implications for contact with the children's birth families. There are indications that some foster carers, although accepting inclusive care arrangements, want this within an exclusive relationship. Social workers need to take account of this.

For the majority of children in public care, fostering is a transitory experience. It is the role of the social worker to keep children in touch with their past and to work for its continuation into the future, and to work with the foster carers to this end. Brannen and colleagues demonstrate that foster children regard their birth families as of central importance and as able to offer 'their only chance of a "proper family"' (2000: 113); these perspectives may not map onto the beliefs of all foster carers. The child welfare service exists to serve children who may therefore be experiencing very difficult paradoxes and ambiguities. Foster families are the social services' preferred substitute care for these children so foster carers are immensely significant.

But if foster carers are defining themselves as moral beings via the children's lives, they are not always viewing the birth parents in a neutral way. There is not a consistent positive belief in the importance of the children's birth families with encouragement to retain, where appropriate, emotional bonds. The foster carer's love is crucial and needs to be so, but this inevitably creates dilemmas.

Life-as-foster-carer is dominated by a set of understandings imposed from the public world into and upon their private world. Home is normally regarded as a refuge from the public sphere but foster carers must accept visitations from the local authority, possibly the child's birth family and other welfare officials. There is also an expectation that social services are notified of any changes in the carer's private, personal life, for example in domestic relationships. As a result this intrusion may in fact militate against those qualities of life that social care staff seek for children and which, originally, the foster families offered. Foster care households are constantly under pressure because of the demands of professional caring and public accountability. Daily life for foster carers is circumscribed by the demands of its bureaucratic context; social services bureaucracy can be experienced as so overwhelming that foster carers can easily become disenchanted.

As previously noted, disenchantment in a hostile world encourages the need for individuals to have a primary meaningful bond. The active creation and sustaining of emotional relationships is central to lives in the personal and family domain; a search for satisfaction and self-fulfilment through emotional connection and communication. Issues of someone 'being there' are crucial to social support. It is by being rooted and attached to someone who is concerned that individual children find their own identities through connectedness. But fostered children are bureaucratised children. They are not freely available and foster carers are reminded of the importance of emotional distance. The social services perspective asserts that 'recognising that the idea that "love is all you need" is out of date',[2] perhaps without appreciating that, for many foster carers, love is absolutely crucial. Thus the foster carer's love, via a particularistic tie, may sometimes be in conflict with their legitimate role, which is to look after a child for a finite length of time, since frequently they want to 'own' the child.

It is therefore essential that the foster carers do not become 'disenchanted' and reliant on their emotional relationship with the foster child. Instead they must know that their concern for, and views about, the children are taken seriously as they work with social care staff towards a common goal. Equality with social workers is not practically possible because legally they, and not the foster carers, have statutory authority and responsibility. Nonetheless foster carers are requesting improved status and respect. This raises important and critical questions concerning the importance of the work that social workers do with foster carers. They need to work in partnership in order to provide properly for the children. To be able to do this social workers must have the abilities and skills to appreciate the lives of foster carers; to help carers to understand and to articulate their emotional needs. Research indicates some uncertainty on the part of social workers in relation to foster carers with children in long-term placements (Schofield and colleagues, 2000). Social workers are reluctant to advise foster carers and feel incompetent about giving guidance on behaviour management. This resonates with the findings of this study which identifies the need for a child welfare service that values its foster carers in order to support and work with them. The gaps in social worker practice that Schofield identifies could detrimentally affect the children. Ominously some foster carers perceive themselves as rescuing children not only from their birth families but also from the social services. In summary, any intrusive, invasive relationship between bureaucracy and the private family is problematic and currently may, inadvertently, be isolating some foster carers so that they seek emotional compensation through public children.

Children are placed with foster carers for their own protection. Child protection is understood to include protecting the identity needs of children, as laid down in both the 1989 Children Act and the European Rights of the Child. Relationships between parents and children are more appropriately construed in terms of love and care rather than rights and duties (Harding, 1991). But foster carers are not parents, even though they offer their families. In the private world of the family, where an ideology of love and care triumphs, a denial of the appropriateness of the concept of rights can lead to injustice and exploitation. It is the right of each child to have information and knowledge of his/her birth family. There may be times when foster carers, because they love the children and wish to save them, may unwittingly undermine the children's loyalty to their birth families. Social workers must understand foster carers and their need to love the children. Loving the fostered child may not fit with the local authority's prescription for 'caring'. This may have the effect, ironically, of heightening the disjunction between the world views of the foster carers and the social services staff.

Conversely, however, it may be difficult for foster carers to care, in a bureaucratically acceptable way, for the children that they need to love. The change of nomenclature (and therefore attitudes) from foster parent to foster carer possibly may have been, paradoxically, at cost both to carer and to child. There may be consequential effects on the quality of their care as foster carers shift their perspectives and their behaviours in order to understand the importance of the birth parents and to ensure that the children retain their connectedness with them. Not offering a particularistic relationship may have detrimental effects upon the fostered children.

Although in most foster families it is predominantly the female carer who takes the lead, it is important to note that 20 male carers were interviewed for this research. Five of the male carers consider themselves as taking the lead role, not always in the daily care of the children, but in all formal negotiations with the social services department. They choose to fulfil the more bureaucratic, if not dominant 'professional' role, within the public domain, as demonstrated in studies on parental involvement in schools (Lareau, 1992). But of particular significance is that all 20 male carers have views about fostering. The majority do not distance themselves but speak about the involvement of their own feelings. They are not solely concerned with their paid employment and their careers; work is important but when making work-related decisions they take into account their caring responsibilities. Although most of them perceive themselves as occupying a supporting role, their lives have been significantly compromised by foster care. Several of them have made employment and social changes, actively adapting work and home lives for the sake of the foster children. None of them suggest that they have done this for birth children. They do this because looking after foster children offers them a special relationship. There is evidence in their interviews of male carers' sense of connectedness with the children and their belief that all foster children need close intimate ties with both female and male carers. There are men who give priority to the care of children.

Male parenting is too often depicted as a social problem; absent fathers, those who work long hours, those who do not support their children or who abuse them. Yet, as these transcripts suggest, they can be a social strength and their role needs to be given greater attention. Some councils may not be recognising the contributions of the men who foster. Their importance and relevance as men-as-foster-carers may be dismissed because local authorities over-focus on the particular ambiguities around the risks of allegations. Dominant ideologies concerning home, family and caring may mean that social services staff automatically relate to female carers to the detriment of both the male carers and the fostered children. It is also possibly more convenient as female carers are more accessible during the bureaucratic working day. But fostering demands flexibility and adaptability from carers; this may have to be mirrored more meaningfully by social care staff and meetings organised for when everyone is available.

Foster carers' own children require more recognition. This study confirms that, in some families, children of foster carers are additionally marginalised by their parents' lives. Local authorities provide a service for all children in need but some are ignoring the needs of 'children who foster'.

The aim of this study has been to bring into the research world the understandings of the foster carers so that they can be seen as people in their own right and therefore as significant participants in research. The account also acknowledges their importance as active agents and recognises their distinctive perspectives. This is essential if foster carers are ever to make their own progressive impact upon public debate regarding the social policy of foster care. The intention has been to understand the many differing perspectives of the foster carers themselves. Much has had to be omitted in an endeavour to explore common themes across a heterogeneous sample, whilst also paying attention to any divergent perspectives. Although the study has demonstrated the pluralities of experiences and meanings, it has also identified some common themes; the overlaying of the imperative of caring and of mothering and, for the carers in this study, that their view of self is crucially bound up with the children. Their statement that they aim to 'save' children by changing them is extremely powerful. Their attachment to the children can prove to be both empowering and disempowering; they may feel powerless but are not always constructed as such by birth parents and the local authorities. Although there is no obligation in the 1989 Children Act for social services staff to work in partnership with foster carers, this study suggests that more attention should be given to this relationship.

This research also addresses Berridge's challenge that 'foster care remains an under-researched provision' (1997: 3). He notes the 'insufficient qualitative research' and a need for 'focusing in detail on the dynamics of foster households . . . in which carers' perspectives (are) explored' (ibid., p. 80). This study contributes to an ongoing process to theorise foster care in order to locate it within the wider frame of reference of the bureaucracy of the social care department. It aims to provide a more coherent description of people's experience as foster carers which reflects their own understandings and in doing so has played a part in giving foster carers a voice.

Appendix A
Pen pictures of the foster carers

Isambard and Olivia Bridges (aged 51 and 49)

Isambard does part-time lecturing and Olivia is a local JP. They have adult birth children and two adopted children. Over 19 years they have fostered 19 children. Isambard is very proactive in formal fostering affairs whilst also being very involved with the day-to-day care of the children.

Arthur and Yvonne Daykin (aged 67 and 68)

Yvonne fostered with her first husband and has experience over 30 years. Arthur is retired. Yvonne has both birth and adopted children from her first marriage. Arthur has no children. She has lost count of the number of teenagers, many with their babies, that she has looked after and prepared for independence. She currently has three.

Ruth Charles (aged 44)

Ruth is divorced with two children, one of whom is still living at home. She has fostered for almost 12 years and looked after some 50 young children (placed before their tenth birthdays). She has two young foster boys.

Brian and Tricia Hale (aged 48 and 47)

Brian works as a chef. They have three birth children and an adopted child. They have fostered for 21 years and cared for 55 children. Brian ensures that his working hours enable him to be at home in order to help Tricia during the day. They have a foster baby with profound disabilities.

Stan and Laura Lewis (aged 54 and 47)

Laura and her siblings had experienced institutional care which she described as abusive. Stan had retired early for health reasons. They have two birth children and either three or four adopted children (they could not remember if the fourth was legally adopted but definitely considered her as 'theirs'). They have fostered 68 children and currently have four long-term teenagers. Current legislation only permits registration for three; there has to be an official 'exemption' for any others.

Ali and Khanm Shah (aged 47 and 45)

Ali and Khanm Shah both came to this country, independently, from Pakistan. He retired from work prematurely because of ill health. They have four children who are all high academic achievers. They have been fostering for almost five years and have cared for about 20 short-term children. They have a four-year-old foster boy.

Stuart and Hanneke Penny (aged early 40s)

Hanneke has two daughters from a previous marriage and together they have a young son. Stuart had a very positive experience in foster care as an adolescent and Hanneke's family had fostered at home in Holland. They commenced with respite care now interspersed with short-term fostering. They have fostered for five years and looked after six children. They are currently giving respite care to two brothers at weekends.

Meg Page (aged 65)

Meg has a married son from her first marriage, and has twice been widowed. She applied to be a foster carer on the death of her second husband. She is on a fee-paying specialist scheme and looks after more challenging teenagers, one at a time, for periods of up to five years. She has cared for four lads and one girl.

Grace Moore (aged 60)

Grace is from the West Indies and had worked all her life in the care sector. She is divorced with four adult daughters. She has been fostering for five years and looked after five children, with a sixth about to arrive.

Clive and Kelly Collings (aged 34 and 37)

Clive is a butcher. Kelly had worked in the care sector. They have no birth children. They have been fostering for seven years and cared for six children (long term) and currently have living with them Nathan, their first foster child, now aged 22, and two younger boys. Kelly is registered on a specialist fee-paying scheme. Clive declined to be interviewed.

John and Ann Field (aged 46 and 42)

John and Ann are both graduates; Ann continues to work from home. Ann's family are Austrian. They have no birth children and inquired about adoption but became long-term permanent carers to two brothers who have been with them for just over six years. They are registered for this placement only, which they refer to as 'quasi-adoption'.

Jackie Rowe (aged late 50s)

As a child Jackie had a very positive experience of foster care. She has four adult children and only her youngest son (aged 26) is still at home. She is divorced. She has been fostering for 19 years and has prepared over 30 young people for independence. She has three at any one time.

Harry and Celia Stevas (aged 40 and 35)

Harry and Celia both came to England from the West Indies to join their respective families. Harry, a machine setter, has always worked at the same factory. They have three children, all in full-time education. They have been fostering for over five years and are registered for children aged under five years. They have three foster children between the ages of nine years and nine months.

Richard and Mary Pole (aged 48 and 45)

Richard and Mary are both self-employed, Richard in the building trade and Mary in the care sector. Richard has an adult daughter from a previous marriage. Mary has no children. They had previous experience on a local authority protected landlady scheme for adolescents but have only been registered as foster carers for a few months. They are currently caring for their fourth child.

Keith and Mandy Grindley (aged late 40s/early 50s)

Keith is in the police force and Mandy is a qualified nurse tutor. They have two adult children. Their first placement, a four-year-old, had been with them only a few weeks.

Alice Dodson (aged 29)

Alice had been widowed for three years and has a four-year-old daughter. She investigated fostering as she had planned to have more children. She is registered for two children under four years of age. Her first toddler had been with her for two weeks.

Margaret Barton, Dick Barton and Simon Martin (aged 72, 42 and 39)

Margaret and her husband had fostered when Dick (their son) was a child. Simon is Dick's cousin. Over the years all three have cared for elderly relatives. Dick considers foster care as his employment, although not on a paid scheme. Simon, who attended a school for children with special needs, is employed as a security guard. Dick is the lead carer of the trio. They are registered for boys aged 16 in order to prepare them for independence and have now had three teenagers over the past two years. They currently have a 16-year-old.

Harold and Kathleen Hawkins (aged 63 and 53)

Harold and Kathleen both have adult children from their first marriages. Harold is a company director of his own successful enterprise. They have just become foster carers and have had their first placement, a six-year-old girl, for four weeks.

Steve and Georgina Radley (aged 29 and 34)

Steve works in IT whilst Georgina is employed locally as a sales manager. Georgina has two daughters from her first marriage. Steve has no children. They commenced fostering less than six months ago, agreeing to give weekend respite care to an eight-year-old boy in boarding school. They then realised that they were expected to cope with the school holidays. Just as they were organising this, the school closed their boarding house, leaving the Radley family to cope with full-time care.

Miranda Fish (aged 30)

Miranda is a single mother with a three-year-old son. Her own parents fostered and Miranda worked in the care sector. Miranda was registered for one child, aged under five. She was waiting to be introduced to a profoundly brain-damaged baby who would be placed with her until an adoption placement was identified.

Alfred and Frances Cole (aged 62 and 56)

Both are graduates with professional careers and had been made redundant within the past 12 months. They have four adult children. They had past experience of looking after teenagers through their church networks. They were registered for either two teenagers, or a mother and baby placement but had not commenced fostering as they were supporting a daughter with ill health. They were fully determined to foster.

Daisy Dousadj (aged 40)

Daisy and her Iranian husband have no birth children. They had looked after a series of single placements for weekend respite. Daisy was waiting to be introduced to a four-year-old girl with serious dietary problems who was likely to be placed for several months. Her husband was working away.

Cyril and Janet Allen (aged 64 and 47)

Janet had been a young single mother. She met and married Cyril when he was widowed with two children. Cyril now works for his son as a lorry driver. They were new to fostering. Their first placement, a boy of seven years, had been with them a matter of weeks.

Gordon and Emma Buchanan (aged 47 and 32)

Gordon had previously been married and has an adult daughter. This is Emma's first marriage and there are no birth children. Gordon had previous careers in the care sector but, at the time of interview, was establishing his own business. Emma is a qualified veterinary nurse. They had been fostering for a few months – first, two brothers for a couple of weeks and now two sisters. Gordon had been fostered as a child and described the experience as very abusive.

Mo and Hope Zazemi (aged mid-40s)

Mo is Iranian. He is a farm manager and Hope is a nursing sister. They have two teenage birth children and foster because Hope wants a larger family. They commenced by doing weekend respite for different children. Lindsey who is profoundly handicapped initially came for weekends (for three years) but is now with them full time.

Mike and Louise Jones (aged 32 and 29)

Mike is employed in the motor sport industry. They have three daughters under ten years. Louise would have liked more children. They had had their first placement, a toddler, for some five months when I first met them.

Lenin (aged late 30s/early 40s)

Lenin is divorced with two children. He is an ex-shop floor trade union convenor, now fully occupied with voluntary work. His ex-wife wrote to the local authority stating that she would not allow the children to stay with him if foster children were present. The social services agree to remove all foster children for school holidays. Lenin provides alternatives to custody for young people bailed by the Youth Court. When interviewed he had had his first boy, aged 14, for only a few days.

Appendix B
Vignettes

Experienced carers were asked in response to each vignette:

1   What should they do?
2   Has anything like this happened to you?

New carers were asked:

1   What should they do?
2   What would you do?

1 Dave and Margaret

Dave and Margaret have two daughters, aged eight and six years. They foster teenagers, on a short-term basis and currently have Zak (14) who is likely to be with them at least a further five months until the end of the school year. Social services need an emergency placement for Katy (14), who was with them for several months a year ago. She fitted in well with the family but was very demanding of individual attention. Katy has especially asked to be looked after by them.

They could squeeze a bed into their daughters' room, but have had experience of 'emergency' placements lasting several months.

2 Mike and Ann

Mike and Ann have two children, Stephen (13) and Jerry (15). They foster under fives. They have had Rachel for 15 months, since she was nine weeks old. She arrived underweight, failing to thrive and clearly neglected. The local authority care plan is that an adoptive family should be found for Rachel. Rachel's mother has visited her many times and Ann is certain that she (Rachel's mother) cannot meet her needs. Rachel's mother is opposing the social services department plan as she wants her back. Ann's evidence to the court is vital for the local authority's application that Rachel be freed for adoption.

Both Ann's boys are playing in a school concert. The night before, Ann gets a message that the barrister needs to see her urgently the next afternoon as she will be needed in court then. This will mean missing the concert.

3 Don and Barbara

Don and Barbara's boys are aged 10, 11 and 13 years. They are fostering Neil who is eight. He has been physically and sexually abused. Against all the odds he has settled well with them and is now accepted at the local school as a full-time pupil, even though he can never be 'reasoned' with. His social worker is delighted, believes that Don and Barbara have wrought a miracle and wants Neil to remain permanently with them.

By chance, Don and Barbara discover that Neil is provoking and bullying their very sensitive 11-year-old. Neil is regularly hitting and punching him. Their son knows that he must not retaliate but his life is being made difficult. Barbara is very committed to Neil who is strongly bonded with her.

4 Chris and Viv

Chris and Viv are delighted when Chris's boss asks them to be godparents to his first child and accept with some pride. When the invitation arrives for the christening it includes their two birth children but not the two foster children, who have been with them for more than three years.

Chris's boss knows that they are foster parents.

5 Jim and Sue

Jim and Sue are hosting a large family ruby wedding anniversary celebration for Sue's parents. They are planning a lunch which will probably last well into the afternoon. All Sue's relatives and their children are coming. It is important for everyone that the day is a success.

Jim's and Sue's current foster child, Kirsty (aged 12), is involved. She is very fond of Sue's parents. A few days before the party Kirsty's parents telephone her and announce that they intend to visit at 3 o'clock on the afternoon of the family celebration. They rarely visit her so she is delighted.

Kirsty's father is an alcoholic. There will be a lot of wine and beer at the party.

6 Pete and Hazel

When, after eight years of marriage, Pete and Hazel found that they could not have children of their own, they decided to foster. They have had sisters, Toyah and Petra, for almost six years. It is a long-term, permanent placement. Toyah has always been very attention seeking. Hazel has invested a lot in them both, Toyah in particular. She loves them dearly.

Recently, Toyah told her social worker that Pete had been 'beating' her. Both girls were removed for the investigation. Pete could not work for anxiety. Hazel could not sleep or eat. Eventually the Child Protection team decided that the allegation was false.

Toyah and Petra telephone Hazel every evening to ask, 'When can we come home?' The social services say that they can return at any time.

Pete says that if they return he will find it difficult not to distance himself from both girls, Toyah in particular. Hazel cannot bear to think of the girls as unhappy.

Notes

Introduction

1 The Fostering Network (2004) *Annual Review*, London.
2 The Fostering Network, formerly the National Foster Care Association (NFCA), is the UK's leading charity for everyone involved with fostering.

1 What do we know about foster carers?

1 Act for the Better Relief of the Parish Poor Children, 7 George III, c.3.
2 The Social Work Research and Development Unit at the University of York (1998) quotes costs of £497 million for 5,000 children in residential care as against £267 million for more than 40,000 children in foster care, i.e. almost 15 times the cost. Hayden *et al.* (1999) suggest the differential to be more than five times but explain that the foster care costs do not include social worker time. Personal social services statistics actuals 2002/3, Chartered Institute of Public Finance and Accountancy, 2004, quote average weekly cost of a residential placement as £2,327 in England, £2,074 in Wales and £1,511 in Scotland. The Fostering Network, 2005 cite the average weekly cost for children in local authority foster care in England as £234 (£12,168 p.a.) but argue that it should be £633 p.w. (£32,916 p.a. in England; £31,460 p.a. in Scotland; £29,120 p.a. in Wales and £31,044 p.a. in Northern Ireland).
3 Also the 2001 Adoption Act.
4 Kin carers have increased from 14 per cent in 1996 to 16 per cent in 2002 (DfES, 2002).
5 The Fostering Network's 2004 autumn survey revealed that 56 per cent of local authorities pay foster care allowances below the recommended minimum for carers to even cover their costs.
6 Safer Care training helps foster carers to look after children who have been abused.
7 Kufeldt, 1989.
8 Throughout the book italic print indicates original emphasis.
9 Studies on male carers by Parker, 1966 and McWhinnie, 1979. Also by Cautley and Aldridge, 1975 who suggest that significant factors for 'successful' male foster carers are not being an eldest child, not having religious parents and perceiving their own fathers as warm and affectionate.

2 Towards a theorising of foster care

1 Many foster carers do continue to care and are seen as offering an additional (usually unpaid) resource because of this (NCB/DoH, 2003; Wade, 1997).

2 See, for example, Windebank, 1999.
3 See also Backett, 1978.
4 See Oakley and Mitchell, 1976.

3 Dealing with dilemmas: private and personal

1 Throughout this book all foster carers' statements are quoted verbatim from the transcripts. Italics indicates original emphasis.
2 Arrangement made by the social worker for children to see members of their birth families.
3 Social worker from the local council who assesses foster carer applicants and supports those who are registered.
4 Throughout the book all bracketed notes in foster carers' quotes are the author's explanations.
5 Respite care is offered to birth families and could be, for example, one weekend each month.
6 For example, for statutory medicals.
7 Hochschild, 1990.
8 For details of the vignettes, see Appendix B.
9 See also Sinclair *et al.*, 2004 and their report that, for one carer, fostering had become more important than her marriage.

4 How foster carers position themselves

1 See Rose (1989).
2 Removal of a child from a situation of conflict for a set amount of time.
3 See also Part (1993) who describes how foster carers' children are never viewed in their own right.
4 Sources: Burgoyne and Clarke (1984); Collier *et al.* (1982); Dalley (1996); Graham (1982); Gubrium and Holstein (1990); Morgan (1975, 1996); Ribbens (1994); Voysey (1975).
5 See Kumar (1997) and Murcott (1983) regarding the cultural symbolism of meals.
6 See Kumar (1997) regarding collective activities and Ribbens (1994) regarding the relevance of games in family life.
7 This is in contrast to the Fostering Network's review (2001) which confirmed other large-scale surveys that 72 per cent of carers felt that they should be paid. Discussion paper (2004) *Fees for Foster Carers*, London, Fostering Network.
8 See Jenkins (1965) and the man who fostered in order to act out the role of the father he had never experienced. Also Nelson (1990b).

5 Having a presence through children

1 See also Butler and Charles, 1999.
2 Professionals working in medical and allied fields have at times questioned the accepted attitude that 'love' is incompatible with a professional role, arguing instead that 'love' is the essence of a healing relationship. See, for example, Siegel, 1986.
3 Ribbens McCarthy *et al.*, 2000.
4 Confirmed by research, Hayden *et al.*, 1999.
5 See Rhodes, 1994.

6 Conclusions

1 But see findings of Sinclair *et al.*, 2004.
2 NFCA (now the Fostering Network) internal memo (1999).

Bibliography

Abel, E. K. and Nelson, M. K. (eds) (1990) *Circles of Care: Work and Identity in Women's Lives*, Albany: State University of New York Press.

Adamson, G. (1973) *The Caretakers*, London: Bookstall Publications.

Aldgate, J. and Hawley, D. (1986) 'Helping foster families through disruption', *Adoption and Fostering*, 10(2), 44–49.

Arber, S. and Gilbert, N. (1989) 'Men: the forgotten carers', *Sociology*, 23(1), 111–118.

Association of Directors of Social Services, (Children and Families Committee) Report (1997) *The Foster Carer Market: a National Perspective*, Ipswich: Suffolk Social Services.

Audit Commission (1985) *Child Care Report*, London: Audit Commission.

Backett, K. (1978) *The Negotiation of Parenthood*, unpublished thesis, University of Edinburgh.

Barnardo's (1996) *Too Much – Too Young: the Failure of Social Policy in Meeting the Needs of Care Leavers*, London: Barnardo's Action on Aftercare Consortium.

Baruch, G. (1981) 'Moral tales: parents' stories of encounters with the health professions', *Sociology of Health and Illness*, 3(3), 275–295.

Bebbington, A. and Miles, J. (1990) 'The supply of foster families for children in care', *British Journal of Social Work*, 20(4), 283–307.

Beck, U. and Beck-Gernsheim, E. (1995) *The Normal Chaos of Love*, Cambridge: Polity Press.

Beck-Gernsheim, E. (1992) 'Everything for the child – for better or worse?' in Bjorneborg, U. (1992) (ed.) *European Parents in the 1990s: Contradictions and Comparisons*, New Brunswick: Transaction Publishers.

—— (1998) 'On the way to a post-familial family: from a community of need to elective affinities', *Theory, Culture and Society*, 15(3–4), 53–70.

Berridge, D. (1997) *Foster Care: a Research Review*, Norwich: TSO.

Berridge, D. and Cleaver, H. (1987) *Foster Home Breakdown*, Oxford: Blackwell.

Boase, T. (2001) 'The baby war', *Sunday Times*, 11/11/2001.

Borchorst, A. (1990) 'Political motherhood and child care policies' in Ungerson, C. (ed.) *Gender Caring: Work and Welfare in Britain and Scandinavia*, Hemel Hempstead: Harvester Wheatsheaf.

Boulton, M. G. (1983) *On Being a Mother: a Study of Women and Pre-school Children*, London: Tavistock.

Bowlby, J. (1953) *Child Care and the Growth of Love*, Harmondsworth: Pelican Books, A271.

Boyden, J. (1990) 'Childhood and the policy makers: a comparative perspective on the globalisation of childhood' in James, A. and Prout, A. (eds) *Constructing and Reconstructing Childhood: Contemporary Issues in the Sociological Study of Childhood*, Lewes, Sussex: Falmer Press.

Brannen, J., Hepinstall, E. and Bhopal, K. (2000) *Connecting Children: Care and Family Life in Later Childhood*, London: Routledge Falmer.

Brannen, J. and O'Brien, M. (1995) Review essay. 'Childhood and the sociological gaze: paradigms and paradoxes', *Sociology*, 29(4), 729–737.

Brittan, A. and Maynard, M. (1984) *Sexism, Racism and Oppression*, New York: Blackwell.

Buchanan, A., Wheal, A., Walder, D., MacDonald, S. and Coker, R. (1993) *Answering Back: Report by Young People being Looked After on The Children Act 1989*, University of Southampton: CEDR.

Bumpass, L. (1990) 'What's happening to the family? Interactions between demographic and institutional change', *Demography*, 27(4), 483–498.

Burgess, R. (1994) 'Scholarship and sponsored research: contradiction, continuum or complementary activity' in Halpin, D. and Troyna, B. (eds) *Researching Education Policy: Ethical and Methodological Issues*, Lewes, Sussex: Falmer Press.

Burgoyne, J. and Clarke, D. (1984) *Making A Go Of It: a Study of Stepfamilies in Sheffield*, London: Routledge and Kegan Paul.

Butler, S. and Charles, M. (1999) 'The tangible and intangible rewards of fostering for carers', *Adoption and Fostering*, 23(3), 48–58.

Cancian, F. M. (1986) 'The feminization of love', *Signs*, 11(4), 692–709.

Caulfield, M. D. (1977) 'Universal sex oppression? A critique from Marxist anthropology' in Nelson, C. and Oleson, V. (eds) *Catalyst*, Nos. 10–11 (Summer), 60–77.

Cautley, P. W. and Aldridge, M. J. (1975) 'Predicting success for new foster parents', *Social Work*, 20: 48–53.

Cheal, D. (1991) *Family and the State of Theory*, Hemel Hempstead: Harvester Wheatsheaf.

Cleaver, H. (2000) *Fostering Family Contact*, London, The Stationery Office.

CM 2184 (198) *Children and Young Persons: The Boarding-Out of Children (Foster Placement) Regulations*, London: HMSO.

Collier, J., Rosaldo, M. Z. and Yanagisako, S. (1982) 'Is there a family? New anthropological views', in Thorne, B. and Yalom, M. (eds) *Rethinking the Family: some Feminist Questions*, New York: Longman.

Colton, M. (1988) *Dimensions of Substitute Child Care: a Comparative Study of Foster and Residential Care Practice*, Aldershot: Avebury.

—— (1989) 'Attitudes of special foster parents and residential staff towards children', *Children and Society*, 3(1), 3–18.

—— (1998) *European Trends in Foster Care*, paper presented to sixth EUSARF Congress, Paris 1998.

Colton, M. and Williams, M. (1997) 'The nature of foster care: international trends', *Adoption and Fostering*, 21(1), 44–49.

—— (eds) (1998) *The World of Foster Care: an International Sourcebook on Foster Care Systems*, London: Arena.

Cunningham, H. (1995) *Children and Childhood in Western Society since 1500*, London: Longman.

Curtis Report (1946) *Report of the Care of Children Committee*, Cmnd 6922, London: HMSO.

Dalley, G. (1996) *Ideologies of Caring: Rethinking Community and Collectivism*, Basingstoke: Macmillan.

Dando, I. and Minty, B. (1987) 'What makes good Foster Parents?', *British Journal of Social Work*, 17: 383–400.

Department for Education and Skills (2002) *The Children Act Report*, Nottingham: DfES Publications.

Department of Health (1991) *The Children Act 1989 Guidance and Regulations: Volume 3, Family Placements*, London: HMSO.

Department of Health, Social Care Group (2000) *Quality Protects: Transforming Children's Service*, London: The Stationery Office.

Department of Health and Social Security (1955) *The Boarding Out of Children Regulations*, HMSO, no. 1377.

Department of Health and Social Security (1976) *Foster Care: A Guide to Practice*, London.

Edwards, R. (1990) 'Connecting method and epistemology: a white woman interviewing black women', *Women's Studies International Forum*, 13: 477–490.

—— (1993) *Mature Women Students: Separating or Connecting Family and Education*, London: Taylor & Francis.

Edwards, R., Gillies, V. and Ribbens, J. (1999) 'Biological parents and social families: legal discourses and everyday understandings of the position of step-parents', *International Journal of Law, Policy and the Family*, 13: 78–105.

Edwards, S. (1980) *More than Parents: a Study of Foster Parents' Experiences in a London Borough, their Stresses and the Part Played by the Support Networks*, unpublished dissertation, Brunel University.

Feree, M. (1985) 'Between two Worlds: German feminist approaches to working class women and work', *Signs*, 10.

Finch, J. and Mason, J. (1993) *Negotiating Family Responsibilities*, London: Routledge.

Fisher, B. (1990) 'Alice in the Human Services: a feminist analysis of women in the caring professions' in Abel, E. K. and Nelson, M. K. (eds) *Circles of Care. Work and Identity in Women's Lives*, Albany: State University of New York Press.

Fisher, B. and Tronto, J. (1990) 'Toward a feminist theory of caring' in Abel, E. K. and Nelson, M. K. (eds) *Circles of Care. Work and Identity in Women's Lives*, Albany: State University of New York Press.

Fostering Network (2004) *Fees for Foster Carers*, Discussion Paper, London: The Fostering Network.

—— (2005) *Foster Care Magazine*, Issue 122, London: The Fostering Network.

Freiburg, A. (1994) 'The path to greater professionalisation in foster care' in Thelen, H. (ed.) *Foster Children in a Changing World: IFCO Conference Papers*, Berlin: Arbeitskreis zur Forderung von Pflegekindern.

Gelder, U. (1998) *Childminding: Does it Work for Women?*, Paper presented to Social Policy Association Annual Conference, University of Lincoln and Humberside, July 1998.

Gibran, K. (1923) *The Prophet*, London: Penguin.

Giddens, A. (1992) *The Transformation of Intimacy: Sexuality, Love and Eroticism in Modern Societies*, Cambridge: Polity Press.

—— (2000) *The Third Way: the Renewal of Social Democracy*, Cambridge: Polity Press.

Gillies, V., Ribbens McCarthy, J. and Holland, J. (2001) '*Pulling Together, Pulling Apart': the Family Lives of Young People*, London: Joseph Rowntree Foundation/ 0Family Policy Studies Centre.

Gilligan, C. (1995) 'Hearing the difference: theorising connection', *Hypatia*, 10(2), 120–127.

Glenn, E. N. (1994) 'Social constructions of mothering: a thematic overview' in Glenn, E. N., Chang, G. and Forcey, L. R. (eds) *Mothering: Ideology, Experience, and Agency*, London: Routledge.

Graham, H. (1982) 'Coping or how mothers are seen and not heard' in Friedman, S. and Sarah, E. (eds) *On the Problem of Men*, London: Women's Press.

—— (1983) 'Caring: a labour of love' in Finch, J. and Groves, D. (eds) *A Labour of Love: Women, Work and Caring*, London: Routledge and Kegan Paul.

—— (1985) 'Providers, negotiators and mediators: women as the hidden carers' in Lewin, E. and Olesen, V. (eds) *Women, Health and Healing*, London: Tavistock.

—— (1991) 'The concept of caring in feminist research: the case of domestic service', *Sociology*, 25(1), 61–78.

Gray, P. G. and Parr, E. A. (1957) *Children in Care and the Recruitment of Foster Parents*, London: COI.

Great Britain: Committee and Allied Personal Social Services (1968) *Report of the Committee on Local Authorities and Allied Personal Social Services*, London: HMSO.

Gubrium, J. and Holstein, J. (1990) *What is Family?*, California: Mayfield Publishing Company.

Hampson, R. B. and Tavormina, J. B. (1980) 'Feedback from the experts: a study of foster mothers', *Social Work* (USA), March 1980: 108–113.

Harding, L. F. (1991) *Perspectives in Child Care Policy*, London: Longman.

Harris, C. C. (1977) 'Changing conceptions of the relation between family and societal form in Western society' in Scase, R. (ed.) *Industrial Society: Class, Cleavage and Control*, London: Allen and Unwin.

Hayden, C., Goddard, J., Gorin, S. and Van Der Spek, N. (1999) *State Child Care*, London: Jessica Kingsley Publishers.

Hendrick, H. (1990) 'Constructions and reconstructions of British childhood: an interpretative survey, 1800 to the present' in James, A. and Prout, A. (eds) *Constructing and Reconstructing Childhood: Contemporary Issues in the Sociological Study of Childhood*, Lewes, Sussex: Falmer Press.

Hochschild, A. (1979) 'Emotion work, feeling rules, and social structure', *American Journal of Sociology*, 85(3), 551–575.

—— (1990) *The Second Shift: Working Parents and the Revolution at Home*, London: Piatkus.

Holman, R. (1975) 'The place of fostering in social work', *British Journal of Social Work*, 5(1), 3–29.

Hood-Williams, J. (1990) 'Patriarchy for children: stability of power relations in children's lives' in Chisholm, L., Buchner, P., Kruger, H.-H. and Brown, P. (eds) *Childhood, Youth and Social Change*, London: Falmer Press.

Ignatieff, M. (1989) 'Citizenship and moral narcissism', *Political Quarterly*, 60: 63–74.

Jagger, A. M. (1983) *Feminist Politics and Human Nature*, New York: Rowman and Allenheld.

Jamieson, L. (1998) *Intimacy: Personal Relationships in Modern Societies*, Cambridge: Polity Press.

Jassal, B. (1981) *Short-term Foster Parents' Reactions to Fostered Children Leaving their Care: a Study of the Intellectual and Emotional Impact of Children Leaving Foster Homes*, unpublished dissertation, Birmingham University.

Jenkins, R. (1965) 'The needs of foster parents', *Case Conference*, 11(7), 211–219.

Jenks, C. (1994) 'Child abuse in the postmodern context: an issue of social identity', *Childhood*, 2: 111–121.

—— (1996) *Childhood*, London: Routledge.

Jones, G. (1995) *Leaving Home*, Milton Keynes: Open University Press.

Jones, G. and Bell, R. (2000) *Balancing Acts: Youth, Parenting and Public Policy*, York: York Publishing Services.

Kirton, D. (2001a) 'Love and money: payment, motivation and the fostering task', *Child and Family Social Work*, 6(3), 199–208.

—— (2001b) 'Family budgets and public money: spending foster payments', *Child and Family Social Work*, 6(4), 305–313.

Knijn, T. and Ungerson, C. (1997) 'Introduction: care work and gender in welfare regimes', *Social Politics*, 4(3), Fall: 323–327.

Kufeldt, K. (1989) 'In care, in contact?' in Hudson, J. and Galway, B. (eds) *The State as Parent: International Research Perspectives on Interventions with Young Persons*, Dordrecht: Kluwer, pp. 335–368.

Kumar, K. (1997) 'Home: the promise and predicament of private life at the end of the twentieth century' in Weintraub, J. and Kumar, K. (eds) *Public and Private in Thought and Practice: Perspectives on a Grand Dichotomy*, Chicago: University of Chicago Press.

Lareau, A. (1992) 'Gender differences in parent involvement in schooling', in Wrigley, J. (ed.) *Education and Gender Equality*, London: Falmer Press.

Leat, D. and Gay, P. (1987) *Paying for Care: a Study of Policy and Practice in Paid Care Schemes*, London: Policy Studies Institute.

Leat, H. (1990) *For Love and Money: the Role of Payment in Encouraging the Provision of Care*, York: Joseph Rowntree Foundation.

Lewis, J. and Datta, J. with Sarre, S. (1999) *Individualism and Commitment in Marriage and Cohabitation*, Research series no. 8/99, London: Lord Chancellor's Department.

Lindsay, M. (1994) 'Towards a theory of "careism": discrimination against young people in care (a discussion paper)', *Seen and Heard*, The Journal of the National Association of Guardians Ad Litem and Reporting Officers, 4, March: 32–36.

Lowe, M. (1994) 'Payments to foster carers in the United Kingdom' in Thelen, H. (ed.) *Foster Children in a Changing World: IFCO Conference Papers*, Berlin, Arbeitskreis zur Forderung von Pflegekindern.

Lynch, K. (1989) 'Solidary labour: its nature and marginalisation', *Sociological Review*, 37(1), 1–14.

McRae, S. (1997) 'Household and labour market change: implications for the growth of inequality in Britain', *British Journal of Sociology*, 48(3), 384–405.

McWhinnie, A. M. (1979) 'Foster parents study', Paper presented at First International Conference on Foster Care, London: NFCA.

Masson, J., Harrison, C. and Pavlovic, A. (eds) (1999) *Lost and Found: Making and Remaking Partnerships with Parents of Children in the Care System*, Aldershot: Ashurst.

Mayall, B. and Foster, M. (1989) *Child Health Care*, Oxford: Heinemann Nursing.

Meyer, C. H. (1985) 'A feminist perspective on foster family care: a redefinition of the categories', *Child Welfare*, V, LXIV: 3.

Moralee, S. (1999) *An Investigation into the Determinants of the Supply of Foster Care in England at Local Authority Level*, unpublished dissertation, York University.

Morgan, D. (1975) *Social Theory and the Family*, London: Routledge and Kegan Paul.

—— (1985) *The Family, Politics and Social Theory*, London: Routledge and Kegan Paul.

—— (1996) *Family Connections*, Cambridge: Polity Press.

Murcott, A. (1983) ' "It's a pleasure to cook for him": food, mealtimes and gender in some South Wales households' in Gamarnikow, E., Morgan, D., Purvis, J. and Taylorson, D. (eds) *The Public and the Private*, Aldershot: Gower.

NCB/Department of Health (2003) 'Choice Protects Conference for Foster Carers', 30 January 2003. Online. Available www.dfes.gov.uk/choiceprotects/bulletins no. 066 (accessed June 2005).

National Foster Care Association (1986) 'Report on London working party on teenage fostering May 1986', *Foster Care*, September 1986.

—— (1987a) *Foster Carers, not Foster Parents*, London: NFCA.

—— (1987b) *Foster Care Charter*, London: NFCA.

—— (1999) *UK National Standards for Foster Care. Code of Practice on the Recruitment, Assessment, Approval, Training, Management and Support of Foster Carers*, London: NFCA.

Neale, B. and Smart, C. (2000) 'Children, money and divorce: caring imperatives and economic imperatives', ESCR Seminar Series: *Parenting, Motherhood and Paid Work: Rationalities and Ambivalences*, Leeds: University of Leeds.

Nelson, M. K. (1989) 'Negotiating care: relations between family day care providers and parents', *Feminist Studies*, 15(1), 7–34.

—— (1990a) 'Mothering others' children: the experiences of family day care providers' in Abel, E. K. and Nelson, M. K. (eds) *Work and Identity in Women's Lives*, Albany: State University of New York Press.

—— (1990b) 'Mothering other's children: the experiences of family day care providers', *Signs*, Spring: 586–605.

—— (1994) 'Family day care providers: dilemmas of daily practice' in Glen, E. N., Chang, G. and Forcey, L. R. (eds) *Mothering: Ideology, Experience and Agency*, London: Routledge.

News in Brief (1998) *Community Care*, 15–16 October.

Newstone, S. (1999) 'Men who foster' in Wheal, A. (ed.) *The Companion to Foster Care*, Lyme Regis: Russell House Publishing.

Oakley, A. (1979) *Becoming a Mother*, Oxford: Martin Robertson.

Oakley, A. and Mitchell, J. (eds) (1976) *The Rights and Wrongs of Women*, London: Penguin.

Oldfield, N. (1997) *The Adequacy of Foster Care Allowances*, Aldershot: Ashgate.

Packman, J. (1993) 'From prevention to partnership: child welfare services across three decades', *Children and Society*, 7(2), 183–195.

Parker, G. (1990) *With Due Care and Attention: a Review of Research on Informal Care*, London: Family Policy Studies Centre.

Parker, R. A. (1966) *Decision in Child Care: a Study of Prediction in Fostering*, London: Allen and Unwin.

—— (1990) *Away from Home: a History of Child Care*, Ilford, Essex: Barnardo's.

Part, D. (1993) 'Fostering as seen by the carers' children', *Adoption and Fostering*, 17(1), 26–31.

Pascall, G. (1997) *Social Policy: a New Feminist Analysis*, London: Routledge.

Peace, S. and Holland, C. (1998) 'Homely residential care: a contradiction in terms?', Paper presented at the Social Policy Annual Conference, Lincoln, July 1998.

Pilcher, J. (1995) *Age and Generation in Modern Britain*, Oxford: OUP.

Rees, J. (1996) 'Children who foster', *Foster Care*, January, 8, London: NFCA.

Report of a Drawing Room Conference on Boarding-Out Pauper Children (1876), London: Longman (report arising from a committee meeting chaired by Charles Trevelyn, 10 June, 1876).

Rhodes, P. (1993) 'Charitable vocation or "proper job"? The role of payment in foster care', *Adoption and Fostering*, 17(1), 8–13.

—— (1994) *'Normal Family Care' and Foster Care: Where are the Boundaries?*, Paper presented to XXXI International Sociological Association (ISM) Committee on Family Research (CFR) Seminar. Children and Families: Research and Policy, April 1994.

—— (1995) 'Charitable vocation or "proper job"? The role of payment in foster care' in Brannen, J. and O'Brien, M. (eds) *Childhood and Parenthood: Proceedings of ISA Committee for Family Research Conference on Children and Families, 1994*, London: Institute of Education.

Ribbens, J. (1992) *Mothers with Young Children: Responsibility With or Without Authority?*, Paper presented to the BSA Annual Conference, April 1992, University of Kent.

—— (1993a) 'Standing by the school gate – the boundaries of maternal authority?' in David, M., Edwards, R., Hughes, M. and Ribbens, J. (eds) *Mothers and Education: Inside Out? Exploring Family – Education Policy and Experience*, Basingstoke: Macmillan.

—— (1993b) 'Having a word with teacher: on-going negotiations across home–school boundaries' in David, M., Edwards, R., Hughes, M. and Ribbens, J. (eds) *Mothers and Education: Inside Out? Exploring Family – Education Policy and Experience*, Basingstoke: Macmillan.

—— (1994) *Mothers and Their Children: a Feminist Sociology of Child Rearing*, London: Sage.

Ribbens McCarthy, J. and Edwards, R. (2002) *Making Families: Moral Tales of Parenting and Step-Parenting*, York: Sociologypress.

Ribbens McCarthy, J., Edwards, R. and Gillies, V. (2000) *Parenting and Step-Parenting: Contemporary Moral Tales*, Oxford Brookes University, Centre for Family and Household Research, Occasional Paper 4.

Rich, A. (1977) *Of Women Born*, London: Virago.

Richards, L. (2000) *Nobody's Home: Dreams and Realities in a New Suburb*, Melbourne: Oxford University Press.

Rose, N. (1989) *Governing the Soul: the Shaping of the Private Self*, London: Routledge.

Rose, S. (1986) 'Sex, class and industrial capitalism', *History Workshop Journal*, 21(1), 113–131.

Rowe, J., Cain, H., Hundleby, M. and Keane, A. (1984) *Long Term Foster Care*, London: Batsford/BAAF.

Ruddick, S. (1983) 'Maternal Thinking' in Treblicot, J. (ed.) *Mothering: Essays in Feminist Theory*, New Jersey: Rowman and Allanheld.

—— (1996) 'Injustice in families: assault and domination' in Shaw, N. E. (ed.) *In the Company of Others: Perspectives on Community, Family and Culture*, Maryland, MA: Rowan and Littlefield Publishing Inc.

Rushton, A. (1989) 'Annotation: Post-placement services for foster and adoptive parents – support, counselling or therapy?', *Journal of Child Psychology and Psychiatry*, 30(2), 197–204.

Saraceno, C. (1984) 'Shifts in public and private boundaries: women as mothers and service workers in Italian daycare', *Feminist Studies*, 10(1), 7–29.

Schofield, G., Beek, M. and Sargent, K. with Thoburn, J. (2000) *Growing up in Foster Care*, London: BAAF.

Sellick, C. (1992) *Supporting Short-term Foster Carers*, Aldershot: Avebury.

—— (1994) 'Foster carers and social services staff working together: support and partnership' in Thelen, H (ed.) *Foster Children in a Changing World: IFCO Conference Papers*, Berlin: Arbeitskreis zur Forderung von Pflegekindern.

Sellick, C. and Thoburn, J. (1997) 'United Kingdom' in Colton, M. and Williams, M. (eds) *The World of Foster Care: an International Sourcebook on Foster Family Care Systems*, London: Arena.

Sellick, C., Thoburn, J. and Philpot, T. (2004) *What Works in Adoption and Foster Care?*, Ilford, Essex: Barnardo's.

Shaw, M. and Hipgrave, T. (1983) *Specialist Fostering*, London: Batsford.

—— (1989a) 'Specialist Fostering 1988 – a research study', *Adoption and Fostering*, 13(3), 17–21.

—— (1989b) 'Young people and their carers in specialist fostering', *Adoption and Fostering*, 13(4), 11–17.

Siegel, B. (1986) *Love, Medicine and Miracles*, London: Rider.

Sinclair, I., Gibbs, I. and Wilson, K. (2004) *Foster Carers: Why They Stay and Why They Go*, London: Jessica Kingsley Publishers.

Sinclair, I., Wilson, K. and Gibbs, I. (2000) *Supporting Foster Placements*, http://www.york.ac.uk/inst/swrdu/projects/fosterplacements (accessed June 2003).

Smart, C. (1997b) 'Children's rights: have carers abandoned values?', *Children and Society*, 11: 3–15.

Smith, B. (1988) 'Something you do for love: the question of money and foster care', *Adoption and Fostering*, 12(4), 34–38.

Social Services Inspectorate (1996) *Inspection of Local Authority Fostering*, London: Department of Health.

Social Services Inspectorate/Office for Standards in Education (1995) *The Education of Children Who Are Looked After by Local Authorities*, London: HMSO.

Stacey, M. and Price, M. (1981) *Women, Politics and Power*, London: Tavistock.

Templeton, T. (2005) 'We are family', *Sunday Observer Magazine*, 28–35, 14 August, 2005.

Thoburn, J. (1995) 'Out of home care for the abused or neglected child: research, planning and practice' in James, A. and Wilson, K. (eds) *The Child Protection Handbook*, London: Bailliere Tindall.

Triseliotis, J. (1989) 'Foster care outcomes: a review of key findings', *Adoption and Fostering*, 3(3), 5–17.

Triseliotis, J., Borland, M. and Hill, M. (1998) *Fostering Good Relations: a Study of Foster Carers in Scotland*, Edinburgh: The Stationery Office.

—— (2000) *Delivering Foster Care*, London: BAAF.

Tronto, J. (1993) *Moral Boundaries: a Political Argument for an Ethic of Care*, London: Routledge.

Twigg, J. (1998) *The Spatial Ordering of Care: Public and Private in Bathing Support at Home*, Paper presented to the Social Policy Association Conference, University of Lincolnshire and Humberside, July.

Ungerson, C. (1983) 'Why do women care?' in Finch, J. and Groves, D. (eds) *A Labour of Love: Women, Work and Caring*, London: Routledge and Kegan Paul.

—— (1987) *Policy is Personal: Sex, Gender and Informal Care*, London: Tavistock.

—— (1990) 'The language of care: crossing the boundaries' in Ungerson, D. (ed.) *Gender and Caring: Work and Welfare in Britain and Scandinavia*, Hemel Hempstead: Harvester Wheatsheaf.

—— (1995) 'Gender, cash and informal care: European perspectives and dilemmas', *Journal of Social Policy*, 24(1), 31–52.

Unrau, Y. (1994) 'Role differentiation between foster parents and treatment foster parents' in McKenzie, B. (ed.) *Current Perspectives on Foster Family Care for Children and Youth*, Ontario: Wall and Emerson Inc.

Utting, W. (1997) *People Like Us: the Report of the Review of the Safeguards for Children Living Away from Home*, Department of Health: The Welsh Office.

Ve, H. (1989) 'The male gender role and responsibility for childcare' in Boh, K., Bak, M., Clason, C., Pankratova, M., Quortrup, J., Sgritta, G. B. and Waerness, K. (eds) *Changing Patterns of European Family Life*, London: Routledge.

Voight, L. (1986) 'Welfare women' in Marchant, H. and Wearing, B. (eds) *Gender Reclaimed: Women in Social Work*, Sydney, NSW: Hale and Iremonger.

Voysey, M. (1975) *A Constant Burden*, London: Routledge and Kegan Paul.

Wade, J. (1997) 'Developing leaving care services: tapping the potential of foster carers', *Adoption and Fostering*, 21(3), 40–49.

Waerness, K. (1987) 'On the rationality of caring' in Sassoon, A. S. (ed.) *Women and the State*, London: Unwin Hyman.

—— (1989) 'Caring' in Boh, K., Bak, M., Clason, C., Pankratova, M., Quortrup, J., Sgritta, G. B. and Waerness, K. (eds) *Changing Patterns of European Family Life*, London: Routledge.

Wakeford, J. (1963) 'Fostering: a sociological perspective', *British Journal of Sociology*, 4(4), 335–346.

Walkover, B. C. (1992) 'The family as an overwrought object of desire' in Rosenwald, G. C. and Ochberg, R. L. (eds) *Storied Lives: the Cultural Politics of Self-understanding*, New Haven: Yale University Press.

Ward, H., Skuse, T. and Munro, E. R. (2005) '"The best of times, the worst of times": young people's views of care and accommodation', *Adoption and Fostering*, 29(1), 8–17.

Warren, D. (1999) 'National Standards in Foster Care' in Wheal, A. (ed.) (1997) *The Companion to Foster Care*, Lyme Regis: Russell House Publishing.

Waterhouse, R. (2000) *Lost in Care: Report of the tribunal of inquiry into the abuse of children in care in the former County Council areas of Gwynedd and Clwyd since 1974*, London: TSO.

Waterhouse, S. (1992) 'How foster carers view contact', *Adoption and Fostering*, 16(2), 42–47.

—— (1997) *The Organisation of Fostering Services: a Study of the Arrangements for the Delivery of Services by Local Authorities in England*, London: NFCA.

Weintraub, J. (1997) 'The theory and politics of the public/private distinction', in Weintraub, J. and Kumar, K. (eds) *Public and Private in Thought and Practice*, Chicago: University of Chicago Press.

Wheal, A. (1999a) *Foster Care – The Way Forward – 'Turning Policy into Best Practice': Conference Resumé*, University of Southampton, 17 September, 1999.

—— (ed.) (1999b) *The Companion to Foster Care*, Lyme Regis: Russell House Publishing.

Windebank, J. (1999) *Gender Divisions of Domestic Labour and Parenting Work among Dual-earner Couples in Differing Welfare Regions: the Case of Britain and France*, Paper presented to ESRC seminar series 'Parenting, Motherhood and Paid Work: Rationality and Ambivalence', Oxford Brookes University, 16–17 September, 1999.

Wrigley, J. (1990) 'Children's caregivers and ideologies of parental inadequacy' in Abel, E. K. and Nelson, M. K. (eds) *Circles of Care: Work and Identity in Women's Lives*, Albany: State University of New York Press.

Zelizer, V. A. (1985) *Pricing the Priceless Child: the Changing Social Value of Children*, New York: Basic Books Inc.

Index